Figure 1b Example of a transfusion management guideline for major haemorrhage

Objective	Action	Notes	Page ref.
Control the bleeding	Early intervention – surgical, endoscopic, radiological	Upper GI tract procedures Interventional radiology	32
Restore circulating volume In patients with major vessel or cardiac injury, it may be appropriate to restrict volume replacement after discussion with surgical team	Insert wide-bore peripheral cannulae Give adequate volumes of crystalloid/blood Aim to maintain normal blood pressure and urine output > 30 ml/hr in adults (or 0.5 ml/kg/hour)	Blood loss is often underestimated Refer to local guidelines for the resuscitation of trauma patients and for red cell transfusion Monitor arterial pressure and CVP if unstable	28
Avoid exacerbating coagulation problems	Keep the patient warm		28
Use laboratory data to guide management	*Request laboratory investigations* FBC, PT, APTT, fibrinogen, blood bank sample, biochemical profile, blood gases Repeat FBC, PT, APTT, fibrinogen every 4 hrs, or after 1/3 blood volume replacement, or after infusion of FFP	Colloid solutions can prolong clotting times Take samples early FFP and platelets may be required before results are available	28
Have blood components available when needed	*Request red cells* Pack volumes range from 180 to 350 ml	RhD positive blood may be used for male or post-menopausal female in emergency Use blood warmer Consider cell salvage	16
	Platelets needed? Anticipate platelet count < 50 × 10⁹/l after 1.5–2 × blood volume replacement *Dose:* 10 ml/kg body weight for a neonate or small child; otherwise one 'adult therapeutic dose' (one pack)	Target platelet count: > 100 × 10⁹/l for multiple/CNS trauma > 75 × 10⁹/l for other situations	29
	FFP needed? Anticipate coagulation factor deficiency after blood loss of 1–1.5 × blood volume Aim for PT and APTT < 1.5 × mean control and fibrinogen > 1.0 g/l Allow for 30 minutes thawing time Dose: 12–15 ml/kg body weight = 1 litre or 4 units for an adult	PT and APTT > 1.5 × mean control correlates with increased surgical bleeding May need to use FFP before laboratory results are available – take sample for PT, APTT, fibrinogen before FFP transfused	29
	Cryoprecipitate needed? To replace fibrinogen and FVIII Aim for fibrinogen > 1.0 g/l Allow for 30 minutes thawing time *Dose:* 2 × 5 donation pools for mid-sized adult	Fibrinogen < 0.5 strongly associated with microvascular bleeding Low fibrinogen prolongs all clotting times (PT and APTT)	29
Recognise and act on complications	Suspect DIC Treat underlying cause	Shock, hypothermia and acidosis increase the risk of haemostatic problems, and are associated with worse outcomes	29
Manage intractable non-surgical bleeding	Consider the use of recombinant factor VIIa		

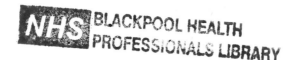

Handbook
of Transfusion
Medicine

Editor D B L McClelland

Lon

Published by TSO (The Stationery Office) and available from:

Online
www.tsoshop.co.uk

Mail, Telephone, Fax & E-mail
TSO
PO Box 29, Norwich, NR3 1GN
Telephone orders/General enquiries: 0870 600 5522
Fax orders: 0870 600 5533
E-mail: customer.services@tso.co.uk
Textphone 0870 240 3701

TSO Shops
123 Kingsway, London, WC2B 6PQ
020 7242 6393 Fax 020 7242 6394

16 Arthur Street, Belfast BT1 4GD
028 9023 8451 Fax 028 9023 5401

71 Lothian Road, Edinburgh EH3 9AZ
0870 606 5566 Fax 0870 606 5588

TSO@Blackwell and other Accredited Agents

First published 2007

ISBN-10 0 11 322677 2
ISBN-13 978 0 11 322677 1

Printed in the United Kingdom by The Stationery Office

Contents

Tables

Figures

Introduction

We have made every effort to include information in this book that we believe reflects best practice at the time of going to press. However, neither the authors, the editors nor the publisher can accept any legal responsibility for any errors or omissions.

More information on many of the topics covered in the book and links to relevant sources are also available on the website **www.transfusionguidelines.org**

We are working with the United Kingdom Blood Transfusion Services' (UKBTS) systematic reviews group to link statements in this handbook to the available evidence. This is an ongoing project and will not alter the fact that there are many areas of practice for which the best evidence is drawn from consensus statements or professional opinions.

This book refers to practices (for example, for blood administration) that, although not supported by reliable evidence from any formal studies, are contained in current manuals and guidelines, presumably because experience over many years justifies the belief that the practice is safe and effective.

Where possible, information about treatment is based on the relevant BCSH guidelines, but in some cases where there is no evidence-based consensus about best practice, the text is based on the practice in a particular hospital and is provided as an example. Where an approved local treatment guideline is available, this should be used. The editors would welcome information from practitioners who have identified and prefer to use alternative practices that have been shown to be safer or more effective.

The manuscript has been widely reviewed by clinical practitioners (see 'Authors and reviewers', page 71) and reflects their comments as far as possible.

New information and correction or amendments to this text will be published at **www.transfusionguidelines.org.uk** Please contact us at this address.

E-Learning resources relating to the content can be found at **www.learnbloodtransfusion.org.uk**

References

For reasons of space, this book does not cite references, but the full text with references, which will be updated periodically, appears at **www.transfusionguidelines.org.uk**

Section 1
General information

Purpose of the handbook

The purpose of this handbook is to help the many staff involved in providing and using blood products to make sure that the right blood product is given to the right patient at the right time. Among those who must cooperate to achieve this are:

- clinical staff who assess the patient and prescribe and order the blood product
- laboratory or pharmacy staff who receive the order and prepare the product
- porters and transport staff who collect and deliver samples to the blood bank and deliver blood to the patient
- nurses and other clinicians who ensure that blood is administered correctly and who observe the patient during and after the transfusion
- phlebotomists and others who obtain and send pre-transfusion samples
- telephone operators who have to make vital contacts in an emergency.

The website **www.learnbloodtransfusion.org.uk** has sections with the key information for these groups of staff.

Terms for blood products

Blood product	Any therapeutic substance prepared from human blood
Blood component	Platelets
	Red cells
	Fresh frozen plasma
	Cryoprecipitate
	White cells
Plasma derivative	Plasma proteins prepared from large pools of human plasma under pharmaceutical manufacturing conditions, e.g. coagulation factors, immunoglobulin, albumin

Clinical governance

The local procedures for prescribing, ordering, collecting, storing and administering blood components should be defined by the local hospital transfusion committee (HTC). These procedures and clinical policies should be based on national guidelines and made readily available to all staff involved in the transfusion process.

New legislation

The UK Blood Safety and Quality Regulations 2005 (BSQR) set legally binding standards for quality and safety in the collection, testing, processing, storage and distribution of human blood components. The regulations affect both the blood services (called 'blood establishments' in the BSQR) and hospital blood banks. For the latter, the provisions include the requirement to show the existence of a comprehensive quality system and the provision of appropriate training for blood bank staff. A record must be maintained of the final fate of each blood component pack, i.e. whether it is transfused to a named recipient, discarded or returned to the supplying blood establishment. Hospitals must submit reports of serious adverse reactions and events to the Medicines and Healthcare products Regulatory Agency (MHRA) and/or the Serious Hazards of Transfusion (SHOT) scheme using the SABRE online reporting system (**www.shotuk.org**).

Guidance on basic standards for clinical transfusion

Standards for transfusion have been developed by NHS Quality Improvement Scotland as a basis for inspection of hospitals in Scotland. Each standard is supported by criteria that can be objectively assessed. These can be found at **www.nhshealthquality.org**

Important changes since the third edition

This edition contains many changes and much new information. Some of the more important additions are described below, but it is emphasised that the following is **not** intended to be an exhaustive list of changes.

New randomised controlled clinical trial findings

Red cell transfusion in premature neonates – liberal or restrictive policy?
The Premature Infants in Need of Transfusion (PINT study) is a recently published randomised controlled clinical trial that has evaluated the outcomes of two different red cell transfusion regimes. Threshold haemoglobin levels for transfusion in both arms of the trial depended on the infants' age. The trial has so far failed to show any evidence that a more liberal transfusion regime was associated with better outcomes.

Fluids for resuscitation – saline or human albumin?
The Saline versus Albumin Fluid Evaluation (SAFE) study was a randomised controlled clinical trial that evaluated the outcomes of resuscitation in critically ill patients using albumin or crystalloid solutions. It found no evidence that albumin was associated with worse outcomes.

Variant Creutzfeldt–Jacob disease (vCJD)
vCJD is believed to be caused by an abnormal variant of normal prion protein that is highly resistant to techniques conventionally used to inactivate micro-organisms. There is evidence to suggest that vCJD can be transmitted by blood and three probable cases of transmission to transfusion recipients have been reported. A wide range of precautions has been introduced to minimise the chance of vCJD transmission by transfusion (see page 64). It has been calculated that if the abnormal prion protein of variant CJD is present in blood, a substantial proportion of the infectivity will be in the plasma. For this reason, precautionary measures in the UK include the use of imported plasma (pathogen reduced) for younger patients; work to minimise plasma content of red cell and platelet components; and numerous initiatives to reduce patients' exposure to blood.

Plasma reduced red cells
The use of this component is mentioned for some specific indications. A plasma reduced red cell unit contains about 100 ml of plasma compared to about 20 ml in a unit of red cells in additive solution. Guidance on the use of plasma reduced red cells has been altered because of the above concerns (see page 55).

Red cell collection by apheresis (red cell component donation)
Automated equipment is being used in some countries to collect a double red cell unit from suitable donors.

Fresh frozen plasma for younger patients
Fresh frozen plasma is now imported to the UK from areas with a low incidence of BSE. This plasma is treated by one of two processes to inactivate or reduce infectivity of any infective agents undetected by testing. The products are described on pages 10 and 12 and the UK Department of Health's policy is that imported, pathogen-reduced plasma should always be used for patients up to 16 years of age (see page 55).

Fresh frozen plasma for treatment of thrombotic thrombocytopenic purpura
Because of the high donor exposure, the UK Department of Health policy is that these patients should be treated with non-UK pathogen-reduced plasma and that, because there is a limited experience of the use of Methylene Blue FFP for this indication, commercially available solvent-detergent FFP should be used.

Prion removal from blood components
Processes have been developed and are under assessment for efficacy and safety.

Blood tests for vCJD infectivity
Under development by several companies. Timescale for availability not yet known.

Recombinant factor VIII and factor IX
In the UK, most young patients with severe haemophilia now receive recombinant factor VIII or IX to reduce the risk of infection resulting from repeated administration of fractionated plasma derivatives (page 39).

Recombinant factor VIIa
This product is licensed for management of haemophilia A or B patients with inhibitors (antibodies to coagulation factors VIII or IX). It is being evaluated in the management of major haemorrhage (page 30).

Cytomegalovirus (CMV) negative and leucodepleted blood components
The residual leucocyte count in blood components is extremely low ($< 5 \times 10^6$ per unit). This reduces the risk of transmission of leucocyte-associated agents such as CMV or HTLV. However, for patients at risk of harm from CMV transmission, some clinicians prefer to request components that are CMV-antibody negative (page 42).

West Nile virus
A mosquito-borne infection mostly affecting North America and causing encephalitis. The virus can be transmitted by blood donated during the viraemic phase. Donors may not give blood in the UK for 28 days after returning from an affected area unless a suitable test is negative. No cases have been transmitted by transfusion in the UK and no infected UK donors have been detected to date.

Bacterial testing
Pre-release testing of platelet concentrates for the presence of bacteria has become a requirement in some countries and has been introduced in some blood services in the UK. This may reduce the small incidence of severe reactions due to bacterial contamination (page 59).

Time limits for infusing red cell units
The recommendations have been altered slightly following a review of the evidence (page 20).

Patient information leaflets
Leaflets with information for patients about the benefits and risks of transfusion are available from the UK blood services. Making these available to patients who may need transfusion can help to meet one of the new legal requirements for patient information.

Management of blood shortages
As part of NHS emergency planning there is a contingency plan to ensure that if available blood stocks fall to very low levels, critical transfusion support remains available to those who most need it.

Reducing blood administration errors
Electronic systems being used in some hospitals can assist safe blood administration by improving identification and checking of patients and blood components.

Perioperative autologous blood donation
This procedure is currently little used in the UK. Centres that wish to undertake it must now register as a blood establishment under the Blood Safety and Quality Regulations 2005.

e-Learning about blood transfusion
To learn more about many of the topics covered in this book, go to
www.learnbloodtransfusion.org.uk

Web-based consultation on the handbook
The text includes many of the points raised by the numerous responses to the web-based consultation that took place in August 2006. However, there were many points on which opinions differed quite markedly, and clearly not all views can be fully reflected here.

New BCSH guidelines published in 2006
The new guidelines are available at **www.bcshguidelines.com** and cover the following topics: alternatives to allogeneic blood transfusion, management of massive blood loss, use of prophylactic anti-D immunoglobulin and blood grouping and antibody testing in pregnancy.

Section 2
Blood products and transfusion procedures

Blood products

Blood is a raw material from which different therapeutic products are made. These are *blood components* (red cell concentrates, platelet concentrates, fresh plasma and cryoprecipitate) and *plasma derivatives* (albumin, coagulation factors and immunoglobulins).

This section summarises the preparation of the different blood products and the steps that are taken to make them safe and effective. Figure 2 illustrates the steps in processing of blood from the donor to the patient.

Blood donation

The medical selection of donors is intended to exclude anyone whose blood might harm the recipient, for example by transmitting infection, or anyone who might possibly be harmed by donating blood. Donors can give 450–500 ml whole blood, generally up to three times per year. Platelets, plasma and red cells can be prepared from whole blood donations or collected by a process called apheresis (or component donation).

Blood component therapy

During the 1980s, the production of factor VIII (antihaemophilic factor) by plasma fractionation was established in the UK. There was a large demand for factor VIII for haemophilia treatment, and the blood services obtained plasma for fractionation by separating it from whole blood donations. This stimulated the introduction of the use of blood component therapy, in which patients are transfused with red cells, plasma or platelets rather than with whole blood. However, after removing the plasma from a unit of donated whole blood, the concentrated (packed) red cells remain as a viscous fluid that is difficult to infuse. Furthermore, the glucose and adenine red cell nutrients are removed so that conditions for red cell storage are not optimal. For these reasons, current practice is to remove all but a few millilitres of the plasma and replace it with a red cell additive solution specifically formulated to support red cell metabolism during storage.

Routine tests on blood donations

Infectious agents

All donations are tested for hepatitis B (surface antigen), HIV (antibody), HTLV (antibody), hepatitis C (antibody and RNA), and syphilis (antibody). Tests for malaria antibodies, T. cruzi antibodies or West Nile virus RNA may be used when travel may have exposed a donor to risk of these infections. Some donations are tested for cytomegalovirus antibody to meet the needs of specific patient groups (page 42). The epidemiology of infections in the population and among donors is monitored in order to inform future testing strategies for further risk reduction.

Blood groups and blood group antibodies

Each donation is tested to determine the ABO and RhD group of the donor's red cells. Group O donors are also tested by the blood services to detect those donations that contain high levels (titres) of anti-A or anti-B antibody.

Manufacture of plasma derivatives

Plasma derivatives are partially purified therapeutic preparations of human plasma proteins that are manufactured in a pharmaceutical process from large volumes of plasma, typically from at least 20,000 individual donations, i.e. about 5,000 kg of plasma. Controlled thawing, addition of ethanol and exposure to varying temperature, pH and ionic strength are combined with filtration, chromatography and centrifugation to separate different groups of proteins. Further purification and virus inactivation steps are carried out. The final products are supplied as solutions or freeze-dried powders. All plasma derivatives licensed in the UK are treated to inactivate viruses. To avoid possible risks of vCJD, since 1999 the UK has imported plasma for fractionation from areas reporting a low incidence of BSE.

Labelling

Blood component labels

The label content is prescribed by the Blood Safety and Quality Regulations 2005 (BSQR). Bar-coded information allows the origins and processing steps of the product to be traced (Figure 3, page 11).

Figure 2 Production of blood components and plasma derivatives

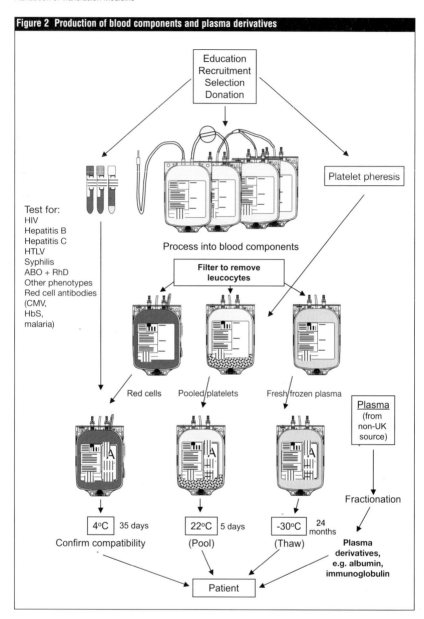

Compatibility labels

Blood components supplied for an individual patient must have a label that is attached to the pack by the hospital blood bank. This label must carry information that uniquely identifies the patient for whom the component has been selected, and may also be designed in order to record the final fate of the component. An essential check before infusing any blood component is to make sure that the details on this compatibility label match exactly with the identity of the patient recorded on the wristband.

Plasma derivative labels

These are licensed pharmaceutical products. The labelling and other information supplied with each vial is specified by the regulatory authority.

Summary information about blood products and haemostatic agents

Table 1 Prescribing and use information common to all blood components

Objective	Note	Page
ABO compatibility	Must be compatible with recipient's ABO type	16
RhD compatibility	RhD negative females with childbearing potential must be given RhD negative red cells or platelets to avoid risk of Rh sensitisation, and should also receive Kell-negative red cells	17, 51
	Desirable that other RhD negative recipients receive RhD negative red cells and platelets	
Compatibility with other red cell antigen systems	Recipients of red cell transfusions must be tested to detect and identify other red cell alloantibodies that could cause adverse reactions: red cells lacking these antigens must be selected by the blood bank	17
Prevent risk of graft-versus-host disease (GvHD)	For patients at risk, cellular blood components must be gamma irradiated	42
Meet special requirements for intrauterine and neonatal transfusions	Specification of components is intended to minimise risks of infectious, immunological and metabolic complications of fetal and neonatal transfusions	55
Ensure that patients receive the correct blood components, correctly administered	Follow local procedures or protocols for ordering and administering blood components Infuse through a blood administration set Record details of each blood component infusion in the patient's case record	18

Blood components

See **www.blood.co.uk/hospitals/products** for a full compendium of information about blood components.

Tables 1–5 provide summary information about each main class of blood product. Details of the quality standards and the manufacture and composition of blood components are prepared by the UK blood services. The blood services' quality assurance procedures are designed to maintain compliance with these specifications. The services are regulated and inspected by the Medicines and Healthcare products Regulatory Agency (MHRA).

Until the late 1970s, most blood was transfused without being further processed to separate plasma or platelets. This blood was termed 'whole blood'. It is now used rarely in current practice in the UK, although in many countries it accounts for most transfusions. Almost all whole blood donations are processed to separate red cells, platelets and plasma. The donor's blood is drawn into a plastic pack containing 63 ml of an anticoagulant-preservative solution, usually Citrate Phosphate Dextrose (CPD) or CPDA$_1$. The citrate binds calcium and acts as an anticoagulant, and the glucose and adenine support red cell metabolism during storage. The whole blood unit is filtered to remove white cells, most of the plasma is removed, and an additive solution is added. To prepare platelet concentrate, the white cell and platelet layer (the so-called buffy coat) is isolated and from this the platelets are separated, pooled and filtered to remove white cells.

Red cells

Red cell transfusion is indicated to increase the oxygen delivering capacity of the blood when acute or chronic anaemia contributes to inadequate oxygen delivery to tissues. The standard red cell component supplied in the UK contains about 20 ml of residual plasma. The rest is replaced by a saline solution containing added adenine, glucose and mannitol. (This is referred to as SAGM, SAGMAN, Adsol or optimal additive solution.) The resulting blood component is officially termed 'red cells, leucocyte-depleted, in additive solution'. In this book, the term 'red cell unit' is used to denote the red cells from one standard blood donation.

Dosage is usually expressed in terms of number of red cell units. This is an unsatisfactory measure due to the variability of the haemoglobin and red cell content of red cell units that is permitted within the current specification (Table 2).

Table 2 Red cells in additive solution

	mean	sd	95%CI	range
Volume ml	282	± 32	284–285	180–350
Haemoglobin g per pack	55	± 8	58–59	35–72
Haematocrit %	57	± 3	54.6–55.1	
Red cells ml per pack	161	± 25		
Plasma ml per pack	17	± 10		4–25
Anticoagulant CPDA1 ml	4			
Additive solution SAGM ml	100			
Storage	Up to 35 days at +2°C to +6°C			
Compatibility requirement	Must be compatible with recipient's ABO (and usually RhD type): page 16			
Dosing guide	Dose of 4 ml/kg (one pack to 70 kg adult) typically raises venous Hb concentration by about 10 g/l Paediatric use (page 54)			
Administration	Use blood administration set; complete the infusion within four hours of removal from controlled temperature storage (page 20)			
Variants	CMV negative (page 42) Irradiated (page 42)			
Cautions	Risks to recipients (page 59)			

Source: NBS and SNBTS routine QA data

Platelets

Platelet transfusions are indicated for the prevention and treatment of haemorrhage in patients with thrombocytopenia or platelet function defects. Platelets for transfusion can be prepared by centrifuging a whole blood donation or collected by the process of plateletpheresis (platelet component donation). In this book the component is termed 'platelet concentrate'. Platelets prepared by each method have similar efficacy, but use of apheresis platelets exposes the recipient to the blood of fewer donors. Currently platelet concentrates contain a substantial volume of plasma, required to maintain platelet function during storage, although the use of platelet additive solutions allows the amount of plasma to be reduced. Platelet function is best maintained by storage at 22°C with agitation. As this temperature favours growth of some bacteria, culture of platelet concentrates prior to release from storage is being introduced to reduce the small risk of a unit being contaminated with bacteria.

The usual dose unit for an adult is referred to as an 'adult dose unit'. It should contain $2.5–3 \times 10^{11}$ platelets. In practice the dose is often defined in terms of the number of whole blood donations (typically four to six) that are pooled to provide the dose. Alternatively a single plateletpheresis procedure can provide an adult dose unit from a single donor.

Pathogen-reduced platelets

Platelet concentrates can be treated to reduce or inactivate microbial infectivity (not vCJD). Clinical trials have indicated that the product is efficacious. This process has not yet been introduced in the UK. A similar process has been developed for red cells, but the product has encountered problems during clinical trials.

Table 3 Platelets

From whole blood donations: platelets from 4 or 5 donations constitute an adult therapeutic dose (ATD)
From apheresis: 1 donor collection provides 1 to 3 adult ATDs

From whole blood (pool of 4 donations is 1 adult dose)	mean	sd	95% CI	range
Number of donors	4			
Volume ml	310	± 33	317–321	250–400
Platelets × 10^9 (at least 240 × 10^9)	330	± 50	329–332	180–400
Plasma ml	250			
Anticoagulant ml	60			
White cells per unit	0.3 × 10^6 per pack			

From apheresis	mean	sd	95% CI	range
Number of donors	1			
Volume ml	215	± 53	206–207	180–300
Platelets × 10^9	290	± 45	289–291	180–400
Plasma ml	180			
Anticoagulant ml	35			
White cells per unit	0.3 × 10^6 per pack			
Storage	5 days at 22 ± 2°C on a special agitator rack (may be extended to 7 days if system is validated and in conjunction with bacterial testing)			
Compatibility requirement	Preferably ABO and RhD identical with patient			
Dosing guide	For a 70 kg adult, 1 adult dose typically gives an immediate rise in platelet count of 20–40 × 10^9 ml			
Administration	Infuse through a standard blood administration set or a platelet infusion set – use a fresh set when administering each infusion of platelets			
Cautions	RhD negative females with potential for childbearing must be given RhD negative platelets to avoid risk of Rh sensitisation (page 17)			
	Plasma in the platelets can cause an ABO incompatibility reaction (page 16), TRALI (page 60) or allergic reaction (page 60)			

Source: NBS and SNBTS QA data

Plasma

Fresh frozen plasma is indicated for treatment of thrombotic thrombocytopenia and for replacement of coagulation factors in a few specific situations. In the UK the only plasma components used are classed as 'fresh frozen plasma' or FFP, although blood banks may now hold a thawed unit of FFP for up to 24 hours.

Plasma infusion was used to treat haemophilia before more concentrated forms of coagulation factor were available. Factor VIII is the only plasma protein of which the biological activity is quality controlled in FFP, although other plasma proteins such as fibrinogen should be present at normal plasma levels. Although FFP is widely used, there are few well-founded indications on which to base a specification to ensure its efficacy.

Pathogen-reduced plasma components

Methylene blue treated FFP (MBFFP) Single donation units are treated with methylene blue and light to reduce microbial infectivity. The level of functional fibrinogen is lower than in standard FFP (60–80%). There are no published studies showing efficacy of MBFFP relative to untreated FFP in treatment of coagulopathy.

Solvent-detergent treated plasma (SDFFP) Prepared from pools of 300–5,000 plasma donations treated with a solvent and detergent. Reduced levels of coagulation factors, protein S and anti-plasmin. Appears to be associated with a lower risk of transfusion-related acute lung

Table 4 Fresh frozen plasma, SDFFP, MBFFP and cryoprecipitate

Fresh frozen plasma	mean	sd	95% CI	range
Number of donors per pack	1			
Volume ml	273	± 17	277–279	240–300
Plasma ml	220			
Anticoagulant ml	50			
Fibrinogen g/l	20–50			
Fibrinogen mg per pack estimated			554–1395	
Factor VIII c IU/ml (in > 75% packs)	> 0.7		1.03 1.06	
Other coagulation factors	variable			
Other plasma proteins	< normal plasma			
Storage	2 years at -30°C			

Methylene blue plasma[1]

Number of donors per pack	1			
Volume ml	232	± 18		
Plasma ml	220			
Anticoagulant ml	50			
Factor VIII c IU/ml (in > 75% packs)	> 0.7			
Storage	2 years at -30°C			

Solvent–detergent plasma[1]

Number of donors per pack	380–2500			
Volume ml	200			
Fibrinogen g/l	27			
Factor VIII c IU/ml (in > 75% packs)	> 0.5			
Storage	1 year at -30°C			

Compatibility	FFP should be ABO compatible to avoid risk of haemolysis caused by donor anti A or anti B
	FFP does not need to be RhD matched
Dosing guide	12–15 ml/kg would typically increase fibrinogen levels by about 1 g/l
Administration	Use standard blood administration set
	Rapid infusion may increase risk of acute reactions
Cautions	Risk of volume overload
	Rapid infusion may increase risk of adverse reaction
Infection risk	Pathogen reduction should reduce any risk due to micro-organisms
	Non-UK plasma should reduce risk of vCJD

Source: NBS and SNBTS QA data

Note:
[1] More detail of SDFFP and MBFFP is available at **www.transfusionguidelines.org.uk**

Figure 3 Blood pack labelling

Compatibility label or tie-on tag

The compatibility label is generated in the hospital transfusion laboratory. It is attached to the blood bag and contains the following patient information: *Surname, First Name(s), Date of Birth, Gender, Hospital Number/Patient Identification Number, Hospital* and *Ward*.
The *blood group, component type* and *date requested* are also included on the label. The *unique donation number* is printed on the compatibility label; this number must match exactly with the number on the blood bag label.

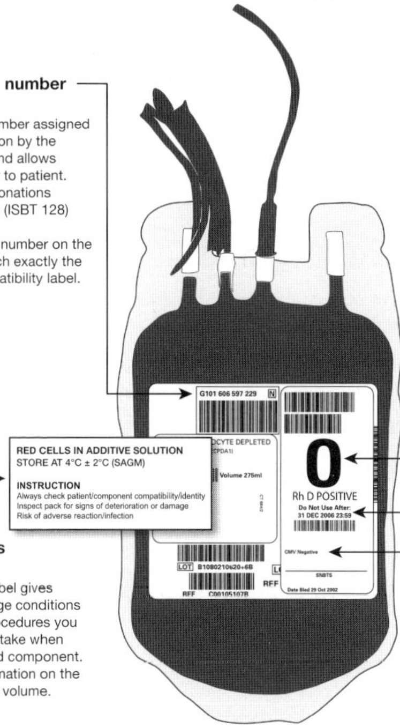

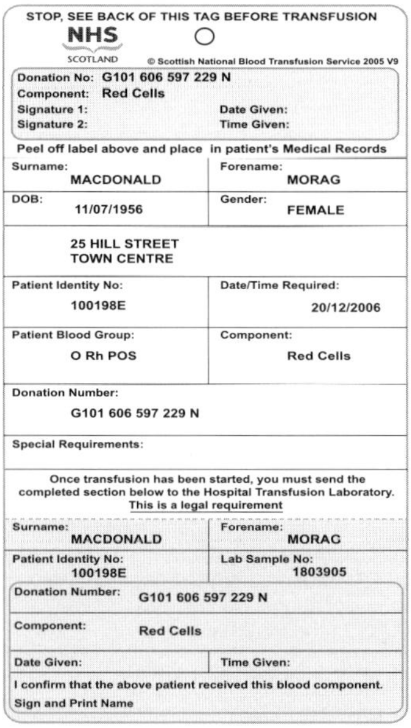

Unique donation number

This is the unique number assigned to each blood donation by the transfusion service and allows follow-up from donor to patient. From April 2001 all donations bear the new 14 digit (ISBT 128) donation number.
The unique donation number on the blood bag must match exactly the number on the compatibility label.

Cautionary notes

This section of the label gives instructions on storage conditions and the checking procedures you are required to undertake when administering a blood component. It also includes information on the component type and volume.

Blood group

Shows the blood group of the component.
This does not have to be identical with the patient's blood group but must be compatible.

Group O patients must receive group O red cells.

Expiry date

The expiry date must be checked – do not use any component that is beyond the expiry date.

Special requirements

This shows the special features of the donation, e.g. CMV negative.

11

injury (TRALI) and allergic reactions. Some clinicians prefer to use SDFFP for plasma exchange treatment of thrombotic thrombocytopaenic purpura (page 45). One SDFFP product, now withdrawn, had levels of protein S below 20% and in the USA was associated with hepatic artery thrombosis in patients undergoing liver surgery. There is a report of late deep-vein thrombosis (DVT) following plasma exchange with SDFFP to treat thrombotic thrombocytopenic purpura. Department of Health policy is now to use SDFFP for TTP. Precautions against thromboembolism are recommended (graduated elastic compression stockings at diagnosis and prophylactic low-molecular-weight heparin once the platelet count rises above $50 \times 10^9/l$).

Cryoprecipitate

Cryoprecipitate was the first practical method of preparing a more concentrated form of anti-haemophiliac factor. It is prepared by controlled thawing of frozen plasma to precipitate high molecular weight proteins, including factor VIIIc, von Willebrand factor and fibrinogen. The cryoprecipitate prepared from a single donor unit contains 80–300 units of factor VIII and von Willebrand factor, and 300–600 mg of fibrinogen in a volume of 20–50 ml. It is a requirement of the BSQR that cryoprecipitate is not pooled in a blood bank unless it is registered as a blood establishment. For this reason, a pre-pooled component (five donor units) is available in some areas.

Dose: A typical adult dose is two five-donor pools (equivalent to 10 single donor units) containing 3–6 g fibrinogen in a volume of 200 to 500 ml. One such treatment administered to an adult would typically raise the plasma fibrinogen level by about 1 g/l.

Granulocyte transfusion

Some clinicians believe that some patients with very low neutrophil counts and intractable sepsis can benefit from infusion of granulocyte concentrates. These may be prepared either by apheresis collections or derived from whole blood. Volunteers for apheresis require premedication with steroids and G-CSF to obtain a high cell count in the collection. Granulocyte concentrates prepared from whole blood donations are also used: doses are lower. Clinical trials have not so far established effectiveness of the treatment.

Labelling of blood components

The blood component pack label contains essential information about the blood component, including its ABO group and Rh type, and the expiry date. Components issued for a patient also have a compatibility label that identifies the patient for whom the blood component has been prepared. This may be an adhesive label, or a tie-on tag, as shown in Figures 3 and 6.

Plasma derivatives

These are licensed pharmaceutical products. Table 5 provides summary information. Product descriptions are available from manufacturers and in the British National Formulary (BNF).

Coagulation factor concentrates

Recombinant factor VIII and factor IX
In the UK, most patients with severe haemophilia now receive recombinant coagulation factor replacement to avoid risks of transmission of virus infections.

Factor VIII concentrate and factor IX concentrate (plasma derived)
Produced by fractionation of large pools of plasma. Current licensed products are all treated to inactivate viral infections and are not reported to transmit hepatitis or HIV. In many parts of the world, cryoprecipitate or plasma are used to treat haemophilia because plasma derivatives are not available or are, like recombinant products, very expensive.

Factor II, VII, IX and X concentrate (prothrombin complex concentrate, PCC: plasma derived)
The main indication is warfarin overdose where there is life-threatening bleeding (page 24). It has been used in patients with haemorrhage, particularly where there is a contraindication to the use of FFP. It has not been tested in clinical trials in this situation. It does not contain factor V or VIII.

Recombinant factor VIIa (NovoSeven®)
This was originally developed for use in haemophilia patients with inhibitors and is licensed for this indication. Other indications for use are still being established. It works by activating coagulation and platelet adhesion, but only if tissue factor is exposed. It requires the presence of platelets and other coagulation factors. Case reports show it can be effective in stopping traumatic, surgical or obstetric haemorrhage, allowing a major bleeding source to be dealt with surgically. The product is not licensed for this indication. There may be risks of thrombotic complications, and as the drug is currently extremely expensive, UK hospitals have special procedures for making it available. It must be used according to local guidelines. Consult hospital blood bank or haematology specialist.

Table 5 Human plasma derivatives

	Human albumin	Human immunoglobulin		Clotting factor concentrates			Others
		Intramuscular	Intravenous	Factor VIII	Factor IX	Prothrombin complex concentrate	
Unit	4.5% solution or 20% solution Various volumes	Varies with product and supplier		Typically 250–1000 iu in each vial			• FEIBA (factor VIII bypassing activity) concentrate
Active constituents include:	Human albumin	Human IgG from a large pool of unselected donors **or** from donors with high levels of anti RhD or anti-viral antibodies	Human IgG from a large pool of unselected donors	Factor VIII: some products contain vWF	Factor IX	Factors II, IX, X; some products contain factor VII	• Factor VII • Antithrombin • Fibrinogen • Fibrin sealant
Other constituents include:	Sodium: 130–150 mmol/ Other plasma proteins Stabiliser varies with product	Other immunoglobulins Other plasma proteins	Other immunoglobulin classes Other plasma proteins Stabilisers vary with product	Other human plasma proteins are present			• vW factor concentrate • Protein C • C1 esterase inhibitor **Recombinant products** Factor VIII, IX, VIIa, activated protein C See suppliers' information
Licensed indications	*Albumin – core SPC covers both 4–5% and 20% products* Restoration and maintenance of circulating blood volume where volume deficiency has been demonstrated and use of a colloid is appropriate.	*IM/SC immunoglobulin – normal* Replacement therapy antibody deficiency syndromes – see page 42. Hepatitis A prophylaxis. Prevention of RhD immunisation in RhD negative women. Page 52.	*IV immunoglobulin* Replacement therapy antibody deficiency syndromes (page 42). Prevention of RhD immunisation in RhD negative women. Page 52. Treatment of immunological disorders. Page 44.	*Factor VIII** Treatment and prophylaxis of bleeding in patients with haemophilia A and von Willebrand disease.	*Factor IX** Treatment and prophylaxis of bleeding in patients with haemophilia B.	*Prothrombin complex concentrate** Treatment and prophylaxis of bleeding in patients with single or multiple congenital deficiencies of factors IX, II or X (and VII), partial or complete reversal of anticoagulant therapy (e.g. reversal of anticoagulant therapy). Page 12, 25.	

Table 5 continues on page 14

TV07403

Table 5 Human plasma derivatives (continued)

| | Human albumin | Human immunoglobulin | | Clotting factor concentrates | | | |
		Intramuscular	Intravenous	Factor VIII	Factor IX	Prothrombin complex concentrate	Others
Prescribing and administration	20% solution: hyperoncotic – risk of fluid overload. 5% solution: use carefully if patient is at risk of sodium retention.	Must never be given by IV route.	Closely observe manufacturer's instructions on infusion rate and dose.	Should be used under the guidance of a specialist clinician.			
Storage	Room temperature.	Follow supplier's instructions.	Follow supplier's instructions.	Follow supplier's instructions.			

Note:
* In the UK, recombinant products are generally used.

Drugs promoting haemostasis

Systemic anti-fibrinolytic agents

Systematic reviews of randomised controlled clinical trials, mainly in cardiac and orthopaedic surgery, indicate that use of these drugs is associated with a reduction in the proportion of patients transfused and the number of units of red cells administered to them.

Tranexamic acid or epsilon-aminocaproic acid

Inhibits fibrinolysis by blocking a lysine-binding site on plasmin. Generally considered contra-indicated where formation of a large insoluble clot is undesirable, e.g. haemorrhage in the bladder. Systematic reviews of clinical trials in cardiac and orthopaedic surgery indicate that tranexamic acid may have similar effectiveness to aprotinin. Tranexamic acid is much cheaper than aprotinin; it is a pure chemical rather than a bovine tissue extract, and is not associated with the risk of allergic reactions.

Dose: In cardiac surgery, a dose of 2 g iv pre-bypass and 2 g iv post-bypass is used in some units. This is not a licensed indication. In other situations with haemorrhage, a dosage of 1 g iv repeated six hourly in adults may help control bleeding (dose frequency must be modified in renal failure). A large multi-country trial of tranexamic acid in the early management of traumatic haemorrhage is in progress: **www.crash2.lshtm.ac.uk**

Aprotinin

A bovine protein that inhibits plasmin and other serine proteases. There is a risk of allergic reaction, especially if the patient has been previously exposed to this foreign protein. The first five millilitres should be infused slowly. Aprotinin reduces allogeneic transfusion requirements in cardiac bypass surgery and is often used where blood losses are predictably high, e.g. repeat operations to replace valves in patients with infective endocarditis. Some clinicians remain concerned about a possible effect on graft patency.

Dose: A single dose of 0.5–1 million Kallikrein Inhibitor Units (50–100 ml) followed by infusion of 0.2 million units (20 ml) per hour may be used. The 'Hammersmith' protocol is widely used for cardiac surgery (two million units bolus followed by 0.5 million units per hour). Two recent reports of risks of aprotinin have been widely challenged. A prospective randomised controlled clinical trial of aprotinin, tranexamic acid and epsilon aminocaproic acid is in progress.

Protamine

Binds and neutralises the acidic heparin molecule. A strongly basic protein prepared from fish sperm. Neutralises unfractionated heparin but low-molecular-weight heparins are only partially neutralised. Protamine also binds to platelets. A fall in platelet count may occur immediately after administration but is usually short lived. Allergic reactions including anaphylaxis are recorded but are rare. The manufacturers recommend caution in those with fish allergy, vasectomy and previous exposure, and in diabetics who have taken the older protamine-containing insulin preparations.

Dose: 1 mg protamine per 100 units heparin. Reduce dose per unit of heparin by 50% for every hour post-heparin administration. If laboratory tests suggest persistence of heparin effect, give a further 50 mg and repeat the laboratory tests.

DDAVP (desmopressin)

Releases stores of factor VIII and von Willebrand factor from endothelial cells and may have other pro-haemostatic effects. In patients who have already lost a large amount of blood its effectiveness may be limited as these stores may be exhausted. DDAVP may also improve platelet function in patients with liver or renal failure. When used in cardiac surgery or von Willebrand's disease, it has been associated with coronary artery thrombosis.

Dose: Typically 0.3 µg/kg given subcutaneously and repeated if necessary at six-hour intervals. It is useful in patients with milder forms of haemophilia and von Willebrand's disease (see page 39).

Local haemostatic agents

Provide a locally administered coagulum.

Applied fibrin

Bovine and/or human origin. Pooled plasma derivatives (e.g Tisseal®).

Spray-on albumin/glutaraldehyde

Bovine origin (Bioglue®).

Local coagulation promoters

Locally applied thrombin (e.g. FloSeal®).
Tranexamic acid. May be useful in nose packs for epistaxis, or orally for gum bleeding, or at surgical site.
Procoagulant swabs, etc. (e.g. Spongestan®).

Basics of red cell immunology and compatibility testing

ABO blood groups and antibodies

There are four different ABO groups, determined by whether or not an individual's red cells carry the A antigen, the B antigen, both A and B, or neither. Normal healthy individuals, from early in childhood, make antibodies against A or B antigens that are not present on their own cells.

People who are group A have anti-B antibody in their plasma.

People who are group B have anti-A antibody.

People who are group O have anti-A and anti-B antibodies.

People who are group AB have neither of these antibodies.

These naturally occurring antibodies are mainly IgM immunoglobulins. They attack and rapidly destroy red cells.

Red cell units are ABO group compatible if the donor red cells are of the identical ABO group to the recipient. Red cell units with a different ABO group from that of the recipient may also be ABO compatible, as shown below.

Patient's ABO blood group	Patient's plasma contains	Red cell units that are compatible
O	Anti A + B	O
A	Anti B	A O
B	Anti A	B O
AB	Neither	A B AB O

Thus group O red cell units can be given to a patient of any ABO group in an urgent situation, as the transfused red cells have no A or B antigens to react with the recipient's antibodies. However, there is a risk of a haemolytic reaction if the patient has antibodies against other red cell antigens. This is most likely if the patient has had pregnancies or has previously been transfused with red cells. In an emergency, the risk of a reaction must be balanced against the risk due to delay in replacing blood loss.

ABO-incompatible red cell transfusion

If red cells of an incompatible ABO group are transfused (and especially if a group O recipient is transfused with group A, B or AB red cells), the *recipient's* IgM anti A, anti B and anti AB bind to the *transfused* red cells. This activates the full complement pathway, causing pores in the red cell membrane and destroying the transfused red cells in the circulation (intravascular haemolysis). The anaphylatoxins C3a and C5a, released by complement activation, will liberate cytokines such as TNF, IL1 and IL8, and stimulate degranulation of mast cells with release of vasoactive mediators. All these substances may lead to inflammation, increased vascular permeability and hypotension, which may in turn cause shock and renal failure. Mediators will also lead to platelet aggregation, lung peribronchial oedema and small muscle contraction. About 20–30% of ABO-incompatible transfusions cause some degree of morbidity, and 5–10% cause or contribute to a patient's death. The main reason for this relatively low morbidity is the lack of potency of ABO antibodies in group A or B subjects; even if the recipient is group O, those who are very young or very old usually have weaker antibodies that do not lead to the activation of large amounts of complement.

Plasma, cryoprecipitate and platelet concentrates – ABO incompatibility

Transfusion of a small volume of ABO-incompatible plasma is unlikely to cause haemolysis in the recipient. However, infusing a unit of plasma (or cryoprecipitate or platelet concentrate) containing a potent anti-A or anti-B antibody may haemolyse the recipient's red cells. Group O plasma and platelet components should only be given to group O recipients.

To learn more, go to **www.learnbloodtransfusion.org.uk** and study Module 2 in Level 2 – Blood component use.

Diagnosis and management of severe acute transfusion reactions

See page 59.

RhD antigen and antibody

In a Caucasian population, about 15% will lack the RhD antigen and are termed RhD negative. The remainder possess the RhD antigen, and are termed RhD positive. Antibodies to the RhD antigen occur only in individuals who are RhD negative, and follow transfusion or pregnancy. Even small amounts of RhD positive cells entering the circulation of an RhD negative person can stimulate the production of antibodies to RhD. These are usually IgG immunoglobulins. If a woman who is RhD negative develops anti RhD antibody during pregnancy, the antibodies cross the placenta. If the foetus is RhD positive the antibodies destroy the foetal red cells. This will cause haemolytic disease of the newborn (HDN). Without effective management, severe anaemia and hyperbilirubinaemia can develop and may result in severe, permanent neurological damage or the baby's death (see page 51).

Females with potential for childbearing who are RhD negative must not be put at risk of sensitisation by transfusion of RhD positive red cells. If for any reason such a transfusion does occur, administration of anti D immunoglobulin may reduce the risk of sensitisation (see page 52).

Other red cell antigen/antibody systems

There are many other antigens on red cells. Transfusion can cause antibodies (alloantibodies) to develop in a recipient if the donor cells express an antigen that the recipient does not posses. Antibodies to red cells are usually detected in patients who have had pregnancies or who have been transfused repeatedly. Some of these antibodies can cause transfusion reactions or damage to the foetus. Before transfusion it is essential to detect potentially harmful antibodies in a patient so that compatible red cells can be selected. It is advisable to avoid transfusion of Kell positive red cells to women of childbearing potential, to avoid risk of HDN due to anti-Kell antibodies.

Compatibility procedures

Group and screen

The patient's blood sample is tested to determine the ABO and RhD type, and to detect red cell antibodies in addition to anti A or anti B that could haemolyse transfused red cells. Provided no such antibodies are present and the patient's sample is held in the laboratory (usually for up to seven days), the blood bank should generally be able to have compatible blood available for collection in 15–30 minutes without the need for a further sample. Check local procedures.

Red cell compatibility testing (crossmatching)

The patient's blood is tested to determine the ABO and RhD type, to detect red cell antibodies that could haemolyse transfused red cells, and to confirm compatibility with each of the units of red cells to be transfused.

Electronic issue (computer crossmatch)

Red cell units that are ABO and RhD compatible can be quickly issued for a patient with no further testing, provided there are procedures in place to ensure that:

- the patient's ABO and RhD type have been tested and also confirmed on a second sample, retested on the first sample, or the patient has been found to be group O in the first instance

- the patient has no irregular red cell antibodies

- the grouping of the blood units is fully reliable

- the identification of the patient and his/her sample is fully reliable

- the patient's previous results can be correctly identified and retrieved.

When a second transfusion is required
A fresh sample must be sent to repeat the tests for antibodies if the patient has already had a red cell transfusion more than three days previously, since new antibodies may be stimulated (or low levels of antibodies boosted) as a result of the initial transfusion.

Selecting the correct blood units
The blood bank will use the test results together with the information provided on the request form to select the correct blood component. Special requirements, such as for gamma-irradiated or CMV-negative components, must be indicated on the request form.

Blood ordering for planned procedure

Maximum surgical blood ordering schedule for red cells (MSBOS)
Many operations rarely need transfusion, so there is no need to test, label and reserve blood. This helps to make best use of a restricted stock of red cells in the blood bank. For procedures where transfusion is rarely required, the group and screen or 'electronic issue' procedures should be used. For procedures that regularly need transfusion, a surgical team should use a standard blood order that reflects the actual use of blood for their own patients undergoing that particular operation. The MSBOS should be reviewed periodically on the basis of internal audit of blood use.

Pretransfusion and transfusion procedures

Right blood, right patient, right time, right place

The steps shown in this section are intended to minimise the risk of a patient receiving a wrong blood component unit or one that arrives too late. Failure to follow these steps led to at least 787 patients receiving the wrong blood transfusion in the UK in the period 2003–2004, contributing to the death of three patients (Table 25): www.shotuk.org/

Inform the patient (or relative)

It is important to explain the proposed transfusion treatment to the patient (or to a responsible person if the patient is unable to communicate), and to record in the case notes that you have done so. The patient or relative may be worried about the risks of transfusion and may wish to know more about the risks, the expected benefits and the possible alternatives to transfusion (Appendix 1). Patient information leaflets are available from the UK blood services. Some patients' religious beliefs preclude transfusion (Appendix 3).

Prescribing blood components for transfusion: responsibilities and records

It is currently a medical responsibility to prescribe blood components or blood products. Before any blood product is administered, the reason for transfusion, the type of blood component or product to be given, and the prescriber's signature must be recorded in the patient's medical record. Accurate documentation of the transfusion episode assists with the investigation of any serious adverse effects of transfusion. The prescriber's signed note in the medical record, detailing the fact that the patient has been given information and that their questions have been answered, may be extremely important in any future medico-legal case.

Infusion rates and times for blood components

For adult patients

Infusion rates and times depend on the individual situation and must be specified by the clinician who orders the transfusion. Use of a suitable infusion pump allows a precise rate to be specified.

Red cells

Rapid infusion may be required – a unit over 5–10 minutes – in managing major haemorrhage, while in a frail elderly patient at risk of circulatory overload, a slow infusion rate is appropriate.

There is extensive experience of safely administering red cell units to stable patients over a period of 90 minutes for each unit.

The infusion of each pack should not take more than four hours (page 20).

Platelets

Platelets have a short storage life and are generally infused in not longer than 30–60 minutes per pack.

Fresh frozen plasma

Rapid infusion may be appropriate when it is given to replace coagulation factors during major haemorrhage. There is anecdotal evidence that acute reactions may be more common with faster rates of administration.

For neonates

Infusion rates and times are critically important. Guidance is given on page 56.

Procedures for ordering blood

Figure 4 Ordering blood and taking samples for the blood bank

Procedure	Good practice points
Fill in the blood request form	*If the patient can't be identified, e.g. in A&E during a major incident:* • *use the emergency identification number and state the patient's gender* • *telephone blood bank for all emergency requests*
Patient ID: • first name(s) • surname • date of birth • gender • patient identification number	
What is being ordered, why, when it is needed: • reason for the request • what type of blood components are required • how much • any special requirements, e.g. gamma irradiated, CMV negative • time needed • deliver to?	• *Tell the blood bank when the blood is actually needed – if in doubt, phone*
Who is ordering: • name of the requesting doctor • contact telephone or page number • signature of the individual who has drawn the blood sample	
TAKE the blood sample The patient must wear an identification wristband with: • first name(s) • surname • date of birth • address (required in some areas) • gender • patient identification number Ask the patient to state their first name, surname and date of birth Confirm this matches the ID on the wristband and the details on the request form Label the sample tube clearly and accurately at the patient's bedside as soon as the sample has been taken	• *Bleed only one patient at a time in order to reduce the risk of a patient identification error* *If the patient can't respond:* • *take the identification information from the wristband* • *Do not use pre-printed labels on sample tubes*
SEND the sample and request form to blood bank Blood bank should reject a request for pretransfusion testing if either the request form or sample tube label is not correctly completed	**Minimum dataset for patient and sample identification:** • **first name(s)** • **surname** • **date of birth** • **address (required in some areas)** • **gender** • **patient identification number**

Pretransfusion checks and administration of blood components

Figure 5 Transfusing blood components

Collect blood component from blood bank lab or refrigerator

- Take a form with the patient's identification details
- Match these with the label on the blood component:
  - first name(s), surname, date of birth, patient identification number, clinical area
- Record:
  - ID of the patient for whom the blood has been collected
  - donation number of the pack
  - date and time of removal
  - name and designation of the person removing
- Repeated for each unit collected
- Repeated for each unit that is returned

Pre-infusion checks

- Has the component been prescribed by a medical practitioner?
- Have special requirements been met, e.g. CMV negative or irradiated blood?
- Check the expiry date and inspect the pack for any signs of discoloration, clumping, leaks, etc.
- Record the patient's temperature, pulse and blood pressure before commencing the transfusion
- Ask the patient to state first name, surname and date of birth
- Check that the ID details match the patient's wristband
- Check that the ID details match the compatibility label on the blood component
- Check that the blood group and donation number on the compatibility label are identical to the blood group and donation number on the blood component label
- Repeat all these checks for each component administered

Transfuse only if the patient can be observed by clinical staff
Record in patient's notes:
- reason for transfusion
- component(s) prescribed
Take and record observations
Avoid transfusion overnight unless clinically essential

Good practice points

Collecting the wrong blood component from the fridge is one of the most common causes of the patient receiving the incorrect transfusion

The person responsible for the transfusion must check that:
- *the reason for the transfusion is recorded in the case notes*
- *the patient has been given information about the transfusion*
- *there is a signature to confirm the pre-transfusion checks have been completed*
- *there is a record of the date and time for the start and completion of each unit transfused*
- *there is a permanent record of the transfusion episode in the patient's permanent medical notes (compatibility report, prescription sheet and nursing observation record)*

The final patient identification check at the bedside is the last opportunity to detect an error

A failure to undertake the formal identity check of the component with the patient at the bedside:
- ***puts the patient at risk***
- ***breaches professional standards and guidelines***

For the unconscious or compromised patient:
- *be extra vigilant when checking the patient ID details against the compatibility label on the blood component*

If a discrepancy is found:
- *DO NOT infuse the blood component*
- *contact the laboratory*
- *resolve the discrepancy*
It may be necessary to:
- *return all components to the laboratory*
- *take and submit a new blood sample*

Infusion times for blood components

Recommendation	Rationale
Red cells 1. Complete the transfusion of the unit within four hours after it is removed from controlled temperature storage (CTS). 2. A red cell unit that has been out of CTS for longer than 30 minutes should not be accepted back into stock by the blood bank, unless there is a validated local procedure to ensure that any unit returned to blood bank stock is suitable for transfusion. 3. Red cell units must not be warmed other than in an approved device, nor left in sunshine or near a heat source.	Once it is out of CTS, the risk of bacterial proliferation increases with time, especially in a warm ambient temperature. Even a short period of exposure to high temperature may be deleterious.
Platelets Start the infusion as soon as possible after the pack is received. Infuse over a period of 30 to 60 minutes. Do not refrigerate platelet packs.	Platelet function decreases during storage. Delay may reduce benefit to the patient. The risk of bacterial proliferation increases with time, especially in a warm ambient temperature. Platelet function is best maintained at 22°C. Do not refrigerate platelet packs.
Plasma Start the infusion as soon as possible after the pack is received. Typical infusion rates: 10–20 ml/Kg/hr. See pages 55 and 56.	Labile coagulation factors decay once plasma is thawed and the risk of bacterial proliferation increases with time, especially in a warm ambient temperature.

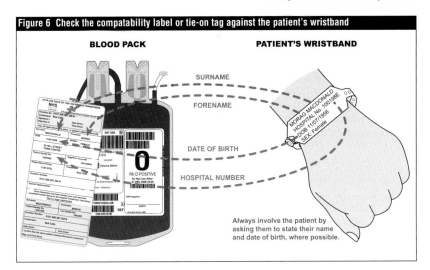

Figure 6 Check the compatability label or tie-on tag against the patient's wristband

BLOOD PACK

PATIENT'S WRISTBAND

SURNAME

FORENAME

DATE OF BIRTH

HOSPITAL NUMBER

Always involve the patient by asking them to state their name and date of birth, where possible.

Blood administration – adult transfusion

Intravenous access

Standard intravenous cannulas are suitable for blood component infusion. All blood components can be slowly infused through small-bore cannulas or butterfly needles, e.g. 21 G. For rapid infusion, large-bore cannulas, e.g. 14 G, are needed. Many transfused patients have venous access established by the use of short-term or indwelling multi-lumen central lines. These are usually suitable for the transfusion of blood components. Where possible, one lumen should be reserved for administering blood components.

Red cells must be transfused through a sterile blood administration set with an integral screen filter (170–200 μm pore size). It is unnecessary to prime the blood administration set with saline. The infusion line should be changed at least every 12 hours and after completion of the prescribed blood transfusion. Platelets and plasma components may be administered through a normal blood administration set or through a platelet/cryoprecipitate administration set. Platelets should not be transfused through an administration set that has previously been used for red cells or other blood components as this may cause aggregation and retention of platelets in the line.

Infusion pumps

There are many manufacturers and types of infusion systems, so it is essential to be familiar with the equipment that is locally available and use it according to manufacturer's instructions. It is essential to use the type of infusion set that is recommended for a particular type of pump.

Rapid infusion devices

Rapid infusion devices that are CE marked may be used when large volumes have to be infused rapidly. Typical devices can infuse from 6 l/hr up to 30 l/hr. Rapid infusers usually incorporate a blood-warming device.

Blood warmers

Hypothermia impairs blood clotting. Studies in surgical patients have found an association between hypothermia at the end of surgery and an increased incidence of post-operative infections and myocardial ischaemia. Hypothermia during surgery should be avoided. Blood and other infused fluids should be warmed. Rapid infusion of cold fluids (> 100 ml/minute) has been reported to cause potentially lethal cardiac arrhythmias. Infusion through a central catheter terminating in or near the right atrium may increase the risk. Only CE-marked commercial blood warmers should be used and the manufacturer's instructions must be strictly followed. Some blood warmers operate at up to 43°C but are safe provided they are used and serviced according to manufacturer's instructions.

Blood must never be warmed in an uncontrolled way (e.g. in a microwave, in hot water, or on a radiator).

Figure 7 Monitoring the patient during transfusion

Procedure	Good practice points
Before starting the infusion • Ensure clinical staff can observe patient • Inform patient to notify staff immediately if they become aware of any reaction • Give the patient a call bell • Record patient's pulse and blood pressure	
Start the infusion and adjust the flow rate	*Observation during and after the transfusion is essential for the early detection of any adverse events or reactions* *Adverse reactions can occur with all blood components and plasma derivatives*
During the transfusion • Record the patient's temperature, pulse and blood pressure 15 minutes *after each unit* has started and according to local procedure • Complete transfusion within four hours of removing the pack from controlled storage	*Additional observations should be made if an adverse reaction is suspected*
If an adverse event or reaction is suspected • Stop the transfusion immediately • Call for medical assistance • Keep the IV cannula open with 0.9% normal saline • Record vital signs including blood pressure and urinary output • Check patient identity against blood component compatibility label • Proceed as described on page 61	*Signs and symptoms of severe adverse reactions often begin in the first 15 minutes of the transfusion:* • *fever* • *flushing* • *urticaria* • *hypotension* • *increasing anxiety/restlessness* • *pain at or near the site of the transfusion* • *loin pain* • *respiratory distress* *Do not ignore any such signs in a patient receiving any blood component* *Transfusion reaction can cause rapid deterioration with hypotension, respiratory distress and collapse*
When the transfusion has been completed • Check the patient's temperature, pulse and blood pressure for each unit transfused • Record the volume of blood transfused • Change the giving set if other intravenous fluids are to be administered or remove the cannula and dispose of the giving set • File transfusion documentation in the patient's notes • If there is no evidence of an adverse reaction, dispose of empty blood packs bags in appropriate clinical waste	*Monitoring the unconscious/compromised or paediatric patient* • *Be alert as they may not be able to report symptoms of a transfusion reaction* • *NEONATES may become hypothermic rather than febrile in response to a transfusion reaction*

Medications

Drugs should not be added to any blood component pack. It is generally advised that an infusion line that is being used for blood should not be used to administer any drug. Dextrose solution (5%) can cause haemolysis and must not be mixed with blood components. Calcium-containing solutions may cause clotting of citrated blood. Use of multi-lumen central lines: page 21. The topics of compatible IV fluids and co-administration of drugs and transfusion are under review by BCSH transfusion task force.

Blood administration equipment for neonatal and paediatric transfusion

See page 54.

Section 3
Clinical transfusion: surgery and critical illness

Good blood management

There are some situations when transfusion is essential, but for many patients the need for transfusion can be reduced or avoided. We have defined good blood management as 'management of the patient at risk of transfusion to minimise the need for allogenic transfusion, without detriment to the outcome'. ·

Who are the patients who are transfused?

Recent surveys of the population that receives red cell transfusions in the UK show that most blood recipients are relatively elderly; many will have cardiovascular disease and may be less tolerant of low haemoglobin levels than younger, fitter patients. It may be unwise to set a very low transfusion threshold for such patients. However, they may also be at greater risk of congestive cardiac failure due to volume overload when blood and other fluids are infused.

Young patients who require transfusion are more at risk of long-term complications, so special attention should be given to minimising the need for transfusion and avoiding known or potential risks. Premature neonates are frequently transfused and are at high risk of identification errors.

Medical or surgical?

This section deals with transfusion of patients seen in the surgical setting. Section 4 (page 35) focuses on the medical context. However, with an ageing population such as that in the UK, many patients who receive blood transfusions have both medical and surgical problems and undergo treatment for both.

Transfusion in major hæmorrhage

See Figure 1a and Figure 1b (inside front cover).

Planned surgery

Blood use varies widely for very similar operations

In planned surgery there are wide variations in the use of blood for the same operations done by different surgical teams. Some units now routinely perform major surgical procedures with little or

Table 6 Outline of perioperative blood management for elective surgery

	Manage haemoglobin level	Manage haemostasis	Blood salvage and transfusion
Preoperative Preadmission clinic assessment	Correct anaemia (see page 24). Increase erythropoiesis with haematinics and epoetin if indicated.	Detect and manage haemostatic defects (see page 24). Stop anti coagulants and anti platelet drugs if safe to do so (see page 25).	Arrange for blood salvage to be available if it is appropriate for the planned operation (see page 27).
During surgery Surgical and anaesthetic techniques	Measured haematocrit or blood loss as a guide to red cell replacement.	Keep the patient warm as cold impairs blood clotting. Rapid haemostasis testing to guide blood component replacement. Antifibrinolytic drug where surgical loss is expected to be high (see page 15).	Intra-operative cell salvage (see page 27).
Post-operative Minimise blood loss and control transfusion	Protocol to guide when haemoglobin should be checked. Minimise blood taken for laboratory samples.		Protocol to trigger re-exploration at specified level of blood loss. Post-operative blood salvage (see page 27). Guideline or protocol specifying blood transfusion thresholds and targets.

no transfusion. This is achieved by a commitment to good blood management, with attention to all the details of the patient's care that together can avoid the need to transfuse. Specific blood-sparing procedures, such as blood salvage, play a part, but their effect on reducing transfusion may be small when the surgical team already practices good blood management. More information on surgical blood conservation can be found at **www.transfusionguidelines.org.uk/**, **www.nataonline.com/** and **www.sabm.org/**

Preoperative management

Anaemia

Haemoglobin in red blood cells carries oxygen around the body and delivers it to tissues and organs. Anaemia is defined as a reduction of haemoglobin concentration, red cell count or packed cell volume to below normal levels. The World Health Organization definition states that anaemia should be considered to exist in adults whose haemoglobin levels are lower than 13 g/100 ml (males) or 12 g/100 ml (females). The US National Cancer Institute considers normal haemoglobin levels to be 12–16 g/100 ml (females) and 14–18 g/100 ml (males).

Patients who are anaemic preoperatively are more likely to be transfused, so it makes sense to try to correct anaemia and iron deficiency preoperatively. For some groups of patients, the impact of this may be limited: in a recent UK study only about 5% of adults awaiting major orthopaedic surgery had microcytic anaemia. A full blood count four to six weeks before the operation allows detection of anaemia in time for the cause to be investigated and for iron replacement to take effect.

Management of iron deficiency anaemia

In anaemia due to iron deficiency, and if there is no sinister underlying cause, ferrous sulphate (conventional dose 200 mg tds: 180 mg of elemental iron) should correct 90% of the deficit in four weeks, whatever the starting haemoglobin. Complete correction takes about six weeks. Iron absorption correlates inversely with ferritin level. Thus, treatment with iron in those without anaemia and with ferritin above 30 mmol/L will have little effect on iron stores. Compliance with oral iron therapy is poor: symptoms attributed to oral iron may be less when the dose of ferrous sulphate is reduced to 200 mg daily.

Bleeding problems (Table 7)

History
A clinical history of abnormal bleeding (tooth extractions, surgery, menorrhagia or a family history of bleeding) should be investigated.

Abnormal coagulation screen
If a patient admitted for elective surgery or an invasive procedure is found to have an abnormal coagulation screen, i.e. prolonged prothrombin time (PT) or activated partial thromboplastin time (APPT) or a low platelet count, the procedure should be postponed while the cause of the abnormality is identified (Table 7). If there is a known or suspected congenital bleeding disorder, the patient must be managed in conjunction with a haemophilia centre: **www.haemophilia.org.uk/**

Low platelet count
Bone marrow aspiration and biopsy may be performed in patients with severe thrombocytopenia without platelet support, providing that adequate surface pressure is applied. For lumbar puncture, epidural anaesthesia, gastroscopy and biopsy, insertion of indwelling lines, transbronchial biopsy, liver biopsy, laparotomy or similar procedures, the platelet count should be raised to at least 50×10^9/l. Infuse immediately before the procedure for optimum effectiveness.

For operations in critical sites such as the brain or eyes, the platelet count should be raised to 100×10^9/l. It should not be assumed that the platelet count will rise just because platelet transfusions are given, and a preoperative platelet count should be checked.

Patients on anticoagulants and antiplatelet agents
Many patients awaiting planned surgery are receiving warfarin or other drugs that affect blood coagulation or platelet function. Where it is safe to do so, it is generally advised that such drugs be stopped prior to major surgery, giving sufficient time for their effect on coagulation to decline. This is an issue on which clinical opinions vary; therefore, patients should be managed according to current hospital protocols. A guide is given in Table 7. More information is available by clicking on the Better Blood Transfusion Toolkit link at **www.transfusionguidelines.org.uk/**

Table 7 Perioperative haemostasis

Management of patients with abnormal coagulation screens, on anticoagulants or antiplatelet medications

Abnormal coagulation screen *Prolonged prothrombin time or activated partial thromboplastin time*	If possible, postpone surgery until the cause of the abnormality is identified.
Known or suspected congenital bleeding disorder	The patient must be managed in conjunction with a haemophilia centre: **www.haemophilia.org**
Low platelet count *Bone marrow aspiration and biopsy*	May be performed in patients with severe thrombocytopenia without platelet support, with adequate local pressure.
Lumbar puncture, epidural anaesthesia, endoscopy and biopsy, surgery in non-critical sites	Count should be raised to at least 50 × 10^9/l. BCSH Guideline for ITP (2003) recommends 80x10^9/l for epidural and spinal anaesthesia in pregnancy.
Operations in critical sites such as the brain or eyes	Count should be raised to 100 × 10^9/l. Platelets should be given immediately before the procedure and the count checked before proceeding.

Medication	Illustrative management plans
Warfarin Options: • Continue warfarin through surgery, e.g. most dental procedures • Reduce/stop until INR acceptable • Stop warfarin until INR normal • Stop and give 'bridging' heparin	In each case, balance the reason for warfarin treatment against the risk of discontinuing warfarin. There are often locally agreed protocols for management of surgery in patients on anticoagulants, and these should be followed. Refer to BCSH Guidelines on oral anticoagulation (www.bcshguidelines.com) and Transfusion Toolkit (www.transfusionguidelines.org). The following are illustrative examples only.
Moderate/high risk of haemorrhage, low risk of thrombosis e.g. lone atrial fibrillation; thrombosis or embolism > 6 months ago	Stop warfarin day 4 pre-op. Check INR day 1. If < 1.3, proceed. If still too high, give oral or IV vitamin K 1–2 mg (depending on INR and size of patient). Repeat INR on day of surgery. Restart warfarin on evening of operation or first post-operative day. Double maintenance dose first day only.
Moderate/high risk of haemorrhage, high risk of thrombosis e.g. mechanical heart valve; thrombosis or embolism < 2 months ago	Stop warfarin day 4 pre-op. Check INR daily and start therapeutic dose of low molecular weight heparin (LMWH) when INR falls below therapeutic range. Give last dose 12–24 hours before surgery. Restart LMWH 12–24 hours post-op when haemostasis secure. Restart warfarin (usual dose) when oral intake possible post-op. Stop LMWH when INR in therapeutic range.
Low risk of haemorrhage, moderate risk of thrombosis e.g. dental procedures, skin biopsy, cataract surgery	Halve normal maintenance dose of warfarin on days 4 to 2 pre-op. Normal dose from day 1 onwards. On day 0 check INR is in surgeon's acceptable range. INR should be in therapeutic range again by day 2 post-op.
Surgery needed in ≥ 6 hours	If no acute bleeding, give vitamin K 1–2 mg iv. Check INR at 6 hours.
Life-threatening bleeding, emergency surgery	Give prothrombin complex (PC) 30–50 units/kg plus vitamin K 1–5 mg iv (dose depending on requirement for continuing anticoagulation and INR). If PC not available, give FFP 15–20 ml/kg (e.g. 4 units in 70 kg adult). Further FFP doses given perioperatively as required.
Unfractionated heparins (UFH)	Stop iv infusion 6 hours before surgery for full reversal.
Low molecular weight heparins (NB prolonged half life in renal failure)	Prophylactic dose: stop 8–12 hours pre-operatively. Therapeutic doses: stop 18–24 hours pre-operatively.
Aspirin* *Even if last dose 5 days ago, consider as a cause of bleeding tendency*	**Preop:** General guidance – stop the drug at least 7 days before planned surgery **but** note that there may be specific reasons for continuing. **Intraop, post-op:** Consider platelet transfusion early in a bleeding patient.
Clopidogrel* *Even if last dose 5 days ago, consider as a cause of bleeding tendency*	**Preop:** General guidance – stop the drug at least 7 days before planned surgery, **but** note that there may be specific reasons for continuing the drug. **Intraop, post-op:** Consider platelet transfusion early in a bleeding patient.
Combination of aspirin and clopidogrel* *Even if last dose 5 days ago, consider as a cause of bleeding tendency*	**Preop:** General guidance – stop the drug at least 7 days before planned surgery, **but** note that there may be specific reasons for continuing the drug. **Intra- or post-op:** Consider platelet transfusion early in a bleeding patient who has been on these two drugs.
Non-steroidal anti-inflammatory agents *Impair platelet function but the effect is reversed when the drug is stopped*	**Preop:** Stop the drugs a few days before surgery if there is no specific indication to continue.

Note:

* A single dose of aspirin (75mg) or clopidogrel causes permanent blockade of platelet receptors and so impairs platelet function for about 5 days.

Preoperative autologous blood donation (PABD)

Some patients can donate their own blood – up to four units – in advance of their own planned operation. It can be stored for up to five weeks in controlled blood bank conditions. PABD may be useful for patients for whom it is difficult to provide compatible donor red cells. It is only practicable if the operation scheduled is likely to need red cell transfusion, if the patient is able to attend to have blood collected, and if the initial haemoglobin concentration is > 100 g/l (female) or > 110 g/l (male). There should be sufficient time before surgery to donate at least two units of blood. The date for surgery must be fixed, so the blood does not become outdated. Iron replacement is required.

UK regulations require that autologous blood units are collected, tested, processed, labelled and stored by a registered blood establishment to the same standard as donor blood. Before retransfusion, autologous units must be ABO and RhD grouped and compatibility checked.

Preoperative donation lowers the patient's haemoglobin level before operation. Administration of epoetin accelerates recovery of haemoglobin after each autologous donation, so that an adult may be able to provide three to five units of blood over about three weeks. Although PABD can reduce the amount of *donor (allogeneic)* red cells transfused, studies show that the *total* number of units of red cells transfused (autologous plus allogeneic) is usually greater in those who predonate blood than in a control group. The use of autologous blood should reduce the risks of developing red cell antibodies and of viral infection; however, it does not reduce the risk of bacterial contamination nor does it exclude a risk of the patient receiving wrong blood due to errors.

Acute normovolaemic haemodilution (ANH)

Several packs of the patient's blood are withdrawn during induction of anaesthesia and replaced with crystalloid or colloid. The patient's fresh collected blood can be re-infused during or immediately after the operation. The effectiveness of the procedure is unproven and it appears to be rarely used in the UK.

Intra- and post-operative management

Thresholds for red cell transfusion in surgery and critical care (Figure 8)

The *critical Hb concentration* is defined as the level below which organ ischaemia occurs due to inadequate delivery of oxygen. This level is different for different organs, but the heart may be most susceptible to very low haemoglobin levels because its basal oxygen extraction is high. On a whole body level, a variety of studies show that the critical Hb level may be about 5 g/dl in healthy adults, children with acute – on chronic anaemia and in elderly patients. In parts of the world where blood for transfusion may be in limited supply or of uncertain safety, clinicians tend to use a Hb level around 5 g/dl as a threshold for transfusing red cells.

Even where blood is safe and readily available, red cell transfusion should be used conservatively in the young because for them it is especially important to avoid any risk of long-term complications, and because young patients without cardiorespiratory problems generally tolerate low Hb levels.

A large randomised clinical trial in critically ill adult patients in Canada evaluated the use of a restrictive transfusion policy (a single unit of red cells when the Hb fell below 70 g/l and maintaining Hb in the range 70–90 g/l) or a liberal policy (transfusing when Hb fell below 100 g/l and maintaining Hb in the range 100–120 g/l) during intensive care treatment. Overall, 30-day mortality was similar in the two groups. However among patients who were less severely ill or were less than 55 years of age, mortality was significantly lower with the restrictive transfusion strategy.

The restrictive red cell transfusion policy appeared to be as effective as (and possibly better than) a liberal transfusion strategy in critically ill patients. Overall, the patients in the liberally transfused group had more cardiac complications, including myocardial infarction, suggesting that anaemia was not a major risk factor for these events. However, in the sub-group of patients who had ischaemic heart disease at study entry, there was a non-significant trend towards better outcomes in the liberally transfused group. Most of these patients had chronic rather than acute cardiac disease. Based on systematic review of this and other smaller trials, current clinical guidelines generally suggest the following.

The safe lower haemoglobin level for patients with acute coronary syndromes is uncertain. A recent observational study suggests that in patients with acute coronary syndrome who develop bleeding, anaemia, or both during their hospital course, early mortality may be higher in patients who were transfused with nadir hematocrit values above 25%. The authors suggest caution in using transfusion to maintain arbitrary hematocrit levels in patients with acute coronary syndromes until evidence from appropriate randomised trials is available.

For patients who are critically ill or undergoing surgery, and who do not have evidence of ischaemic heart disease, a haemoglobin concentration of 70 g/l is a reasonable threshold for transfusion. For those with evidence of ischaemic heart disease it may be safer to maintain the haemoglobin concentration at 90–100 g/l (see also page 32).

Intra- and post-operative blood conservation

Intra-operative blood salvage

Blood aspirated from the operative field can be re-infused to the patient. Blood may be returned as collected or it may be processed to remove plasma constituents. If large volumes of shed blood are returned without processing, the patient may experience coagulation problems that could cause more bleeding. Blood salvage procedures have been evaluated by clinical trials in cardiac and orthopaedic surgery; systematic reviews of these studies indicate that salvage can reduce the proportion of patients who receive allogeneic red cell transfusion in orthopaedic surgery. In cardiac surgery, trials show only a slight reduction in transfusion of allogeneic red cells. This may be due to the inclusion of trials in which unprocessed blood was re-infused. It should be noted that, although unproven by clinical trials, many clinicians believe that patients with major surgical blood losses do better when salvaged blood is reinfused to reduce transfusion requirements.

Post-operative blood salvage

Blood from wound drains can be collected and re-infused using special equipment. This procedure is used in the belief that it can reduce transfusion requirements in some operations such as knee replacement. The re-infusion of unprocessed blood from wound drains may cause coagulation problems, so some authorities recommend that blood is processed by washing before it is re-infused. The effectiveness of this procedure in reducing allogeneic transfusion has not been proven by adequate clinical trials.

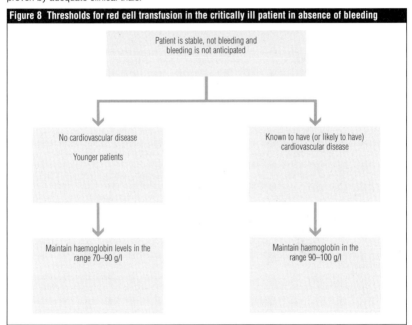

Figure 8 Thresholds for red cell transfusion in the critically ill patient in absence of bleeding

Patient is stable, not bleeding and bleeding is not anticipated

No cardiovascular disease

Younger patients

Known to have (or likely to have) cardiovascular disease

Maintain haemoglobin levels in the range 70–90 g/l

Maintain haemoglobin in the range 90–100 g/l

Post-operative anaemia

After a major operation, provided iron stores are adequate and the patient has normal bone marrow function, the reticulocyte count begins to rise after a week or so and by one month after operation, about 60% of the perioperative fall in haemoglobin will typically have been regained.

Iron stores equivalent to a ferritin of 15–20 micromol/l are required for each gram/dl of haemoglobin recovered. Post-operatively, many patients become iron deficient as a result of the operative blood loss and utilisation of iron stores for recovery.

Management: Iron given preoperatively is only likely to be effective if the patient's iron stores are low (ferritin below 30 micromol/l). Post-operatively, absorption of iron is probably good in patients without other chronic disease.

A three to four week course of iron supplements started on post-operative day seven should be considered for a patient with low preoperative iron stores and large perioperative loss of haemoglobin. (See page 35 – oral iron replacement.)

Major haemorrhage: surgery, trauma, obstetrics and gastrointestinal

This section gives general guidance about transfusion management of a bleeding patient who is likely to need rapid infusion of substantial volumes of fluid together with red cell replacement, sometimes referred to as massive haemorrhage. (See also obstetric haemorrhage, page 51 and gastrointestinal haemorrhage, page 32.) See also the 2006 BCSH Guideline.

Fluid resuscitation

Systematic reviews reveal uncertainty about the best approach to restoration of circulating volume in hypovolaemic shock. Full restoration of volume may worsen bleeding by increasing blood pressure and diluting clotting factors in the blood. Some patients, e.g. those with ruptured aortic aneurysm or blunt chest trauma, do not benefit from full restoration of blood volume and blood pressure before surgical control of bleeding. However, with severe head injuries, restoration of blood volume and pressure may reduce the extent of ischaemic brain damage.

A recent randomised controlled trial of 5% human albumin vs saline infusion showed in a hetero-geneous population of adult ICU patients that albumin can be considered safe, without demon-strating any clear efficacy advantage over saline. There is no firm evidence that the use of any col-loid solution is superior to any other or that colloid solutions are associated with better outcomes than crystalloids in patients with trauma or burns or following surgery. Some colloid solutions affect haemostatic function and so could contribute to a bleeding tendency. It is advisable to adhere to the maximum doses recommend by the manufacturers.

Clinical and laboratory evidence of coagulopathy

Microvascular bleeding
This term describes a condition following major blood loss in which there is abnormal bleeding with oozing from tissues and puncture sites in a patient who has major bleeding, clotting problems resulting from dilution and/or consumption of platelets and coagulation factors.

Dilutional coagulopathy
Fibrinogen concentration halves after every 0.75 blood volume replaced. As a rough guide it is likely to fall to < 1 g/l after replacement of 12 units of red cells or 1.5 × blood volume. Other clotting fac-tors fall by varying degrees because some, such as factor IX, have considerable extravascular dis-tribution, whereas factor VIII is largely intravascular but is released from endothelial cells at times of stress. As a guide, when red cells in additive solution are transfused, a prothrombin time ratio (PTR) of > 1.5 (clotting factors approximately 50% of normal) will be reached after replacement of 1–1.5 × blood volume, or transfusion of 8–12 units of red cells. A PTR of > 1.8 (clotting factors approximately 30% of normal) will be reached after replacement of 2 × blood volume. Platelet count will halve for every 1 × blood volume replaced and, depending on the starting count, will usually fall to 50–100 × 10^9/l after 2 × blood volume replacement, or transfusion of > 15 units of red cells.

Disseminated intravascular coagulation
Acute disseminated intravascular coagulation (DIC) results from activation of the coagulation and fibrinolytic systems leading to consumption of platelets, coagulation proteins, fibrinogen and platelets. It is most often seen in patients with sepsis or an obstetric complication. There may be severe microvascular bleeding with or without thrombotic complications. DIC may be provoked by tissue damage due to trauma or by underperfusion, hypothermia, sepsis or obstetric complications. Diagnosis is by clinical signs of unexpected bleeding or thrombosis, low fibrinogen or platelets, prolonged PTR and raised fibrin degradation products (FDP) or d-dimers.

Hypothermia, acidosis, hypocalcaemia in massive haemorrhage
May occur during haemorrhage and resuscitation and must be corrected as they contribute to the bleeding tendency. See Table 8.

Blood salvage (cell salvage)
May be an important contribution to management in some cases of major haemorrhage (page 27).

Table 8 Other complications of large-volume transfusions

Problem	Prevention/treatment
Hypothermia coagulopathy and O_2 delivery Hypothermia impairs haemostasis and shifts the Bohr curve to the left, reducing red cell oxygen delivery to the tissues. Rapid transfusion of blood at 4°C can lower the core temperature by several degrees.	Keep the patient warm.
Hypocalcaemia FFP or platelets contain citrate anticoagulant (red cells in additive solution contain only traces of citrate). In theory, infused citrate could lower plasma ionised calcium levels, but in adults rapid liver metabolism of citrate usually prevents this. In neonates and patients who are hypothermic, the combined effects of hypocalcaemia and hyperkalaemia may be cardiotoxic.	If there is ECG or clinical evidence of hypocalcaemia, give 5 ml of 10% calcium gluconate (for an adult) by *slow* IV injection and, if necessary, repeated until the ECG is normal. *It is very unusual for IV calcium to be needed during blood component transfusion.*
Hyperkalaemia The plasma or additive solution in a unit of red cells stored for 4–5 weeks may contain 5–10 mmol of potassium. In the presence of acidaema and hypothermia, this additional potassium can lead to cardiac arrest.	Keep the patient warm and monitor potassium levels during massive transfusion.
Acid-base disturbance Despite the lactic acid content of transfused blood (1–2 mmol/unit of red cells, 3–10 mmol/unit of whole blood), fluid resuscitation usually improves acidosis in a shocked patient. Transfused citrate can contribute to metabolic alkalosis when large volumes of blood components are infused.	
Adult respiratory distress syndrome 1. Due to large volume transfusion. 2. Transfusion-related acute-lung injury (TRALI) due to reaction with antibodies in a single plasma-containing component should be considered (see page 60).	The risk is minimised if good perfusion and oxygenation are maintained and over-transfusion is avoided. Monitor appropriately. Treat with oxygen, positive end-expiratory pressure and mechanical ventilation. Beware of sudden systemic hypovolaemia with TRALI.

Use of blood components in the patient who is bleeding (Table 9)

The statements in the following section reflect current clinical guidelines and the views of clinicians with relevant clinical experience.

In a patient *who is bleeding* and has evidence of a coagulopathy (or is likely to develop a coagulopathy), it is sensible to give blood components *before* coagulation deteriorates and worsens the bleeding.

If the major source of bleeding has been controlled and there is no microvascular bleeding, there is no need to give blood components even if laboratory coagulation tests are abnormal.

Table 9 Use of blood components in the patient who is bleeding

Product	Indication and target levels	Dose
Fresh frozen plasma *30 minutes to thaw*	Dilutional coagulopathy with a PTR greater than 1.5 is likely after replacement of 1–1.5 blood volumes within six hours. If bleeding continues, FFP may avoid a worsening coagulopathy and bleeding from the primary source, but it will not stop the primary cause of the bleeding.	An initial dose of 15 ml/kg is generally recommended (four or five donor units of FFP). Further doses should only be given if bleeding continues and should be guided by the prothrombin time and activated partial thromboplastin time (APTT).
Cryoprecipitate *30 minutes to thaw*	May be indicated when there is bleeding with a fibrinogen concentration below 1 g/l.	Two pooled units equivalent to 10 single donor units: 3–6 g fibrinogen in 200 to 500 ml should raise the plasma fibrinogen level in an adult by about 1 g/l (see Table 4).
Platelet concentrate *Check delivery delay: may need to be transported from blood centre*	Platelet count is unlikely to fall below a critical level of 50×10^9/l until 1.5–2.5 blood volumes have been replaced. Count should be maintained above 75×10^9/l. In multiple or CNS trauma above 100×10^9/l.	Adult dose unit: $2.5–3 \times 10^{11}$ platelets should raise the platelet count by about 50×10^9/l, but less in consumptive coagulopathy, e.g. DIC. If bleeding continues, monitor the platelet count as further transfusion may be needed to maintain target count.

Recombinant factor VIIa (NovoSeven®) in haemorrhage

Criteria for use may include severe haemorrhage where there is a reasonable prospect of long-term recovery, e.g. multiple trauma, focal bleeding points have been dealt with and effective replacement of coagulation factors and platelets has been shown by laboratory tests (e.g. fibrinogen > 1 g, platelets > 50 PTR < 1.8).

Other adverse factors such as heparin, hypothermia, acidosis, hypocalcaemia, etc. should have been excluded or corrected, other available interventions, such as an antibrinolytic and local haemostatic agents, have been used, and the risk of thrombosis in critical small vessel anastomoses has been assessed.

Randomised controlled clinical trials have not yet established clear indications for recombinant factor VIIa in haemorrhage other than in some patients with intracranial haemorrhage.

Dose: Typical dose schedule is 90 micrograms/kg rounded up to a whole vial. Repeat at three hours if necessary.

Note: NovoSeven® is not licensed in the UK for this indication. Local procedures for documenting its use must be followed.

Anticipated massive transfusion

Patients such as those with ruptured aortic aneurysms often develop DIC as well as dilutional coagulopathy due to fluid resuscitation. Early administration of FFP may help to avoid this. The risks of administering FFP are likely to be small in relation to the patient's overall risks and prognosis. Such use should be according to locally developed protocols that specify regular monitoring of coagulation.

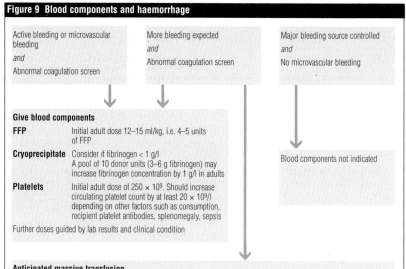

Figure 9 Blood components and haemorrhage

Active bleeding or microvascular bleeding
and
Abnormal coagulation screen

More bleeding expected
and
Abnormal coagulation screen

Major bleeding source controlled
and
No microvascular bleeding

Give blood components

FFP — Initial adult dose 12–15 ml/kg, i.e. 4–5 units of FFP

Cryoprecipitate — Consider if fibrinogen < 1 g/l
A pool of 10 donor units (3–6 g fibrinogen) may increase fibrinogen concentration by 1 g/l in adults

Platelets — Initial adult dose of 250 × 10⁹. Should increase circulating platelet count by at least 20 × 10⁹/l depending on other factors such as consumption, recipient platelet antibodies, splenomegaly, sepsis

Further doses guided by lab results and clinical condition

Blood components not indicated

Anticipated massive transfusion

In patients such as those with ruptured aortic aneurysms there is often a severe consumption coagulopathy in addition to the dilutional coagulopathy associated with fluid resuscitation.

It may be prudent practice to give FFP at an early stage to avoid the added complication of the development of dilutional coagulopathy. The risks and costs of FFP used in this way are small compared to the risk of death or major morbidity from the patients presenting problems. Such use should be according to locally developed protocols that specify regular monitoring of the coagulation screen.

Management of a bleeding patient who has received fibrinolytics or platelet inhibitors

Systemic fibrinolytics (Table 7)

These work by activating plasminogen to plasmin, and reducing or saturating anti-plasmin (t1/2 = 2.5 days). Streptokinase has a variable plasma half-life depending on anti-streptokinase antibody levels. Recombinant tissue plasminogen activator (Alteplase) has a plasma half-life of four to five minutes only, but there is a smaller tissue pool with a half-life of about 40 minutes. Anti-plasmin levels and plasminogen levels will increase after cessation of treatment. Fibrinogen levels may decrease markedly, particularly after streptokinase.

Management: Active treatment of haemorrhage, or preparation for emergency surgery, may include anti-fibrinolytic agents (e.g. aprotinin or tranexamic acid) and cryoprecipitate/FFP to restore reduced fibrinogen levels. The fibrinolytic activity of these drugs should be minimal a couple of hours after cessation of treatment, but reduced levels of plasmin, anti-plasmin and fibrinogen may persist for longer.

Aspirin or clopidogrel

Platelet inhibition by either one of these drugs alone will produce a small increase in clinical bleeding time.

Management: No specific action is needed but in a patient on either of these drugs who is bleeding, platelet transfusion may be considered even with a normal or moderately reduced platelet count.

Aspirin and clopidogrel

Used together, these drugs result in a much more clinically significant platelet defect. Both agents block platelet receptors permanently (platelet lifespan = 10 days). Even if the last dose was given as long as five days ago, these drugs should still be considered as a cause of bleeding tendency.

Management: Platelet transfusion should be considered early in bleeding patients who have been on this combination of drugs.

Inhibitors of platelet surface receptors GPIIb/IIIa

High-avidity agents such as Abciximab
These bind strongly to platelet receptors and inhibit platelet function for 12–24 hours, but little active drug remains in the plasma at two hours after administration.

Management: The drug effect can be partially reversed by platelet transfusion.

Low-molecular-weight agents (e.g. Eptifibatide, Tirofiban)
These bind reversibly to platelet receptors and will also bind donor platelet receptors. The half-life of these agents is short (1.5–2.5 hours) and the effect on the patient's own platelets should reverse over a few hours.

Management: Platelet transfusion will be of little benefit in the absence of thrombocytopenia.

Cardiac surgery

Cardiopulmonary bypass during cardiac surgery can impair haemostasis and contribute to bleeding. There is no evidence that prophylactic use of FFP, cryoprecipitate and platelets reduces bleeding, but blood components may be used to correct dilutional coagulopathy consequent on blood loss. Platelets are frequently used but with modern bypass methods there is no evidence to show any benefit in the absence of significant thrombocytopenia or a specific platelet defect. Antifibrinolytic agents (aprotinin and tranexamic acid) have been consistently shown to reduce blood loss in cardiac surgery in both high-risk and routine patients. Aprotinin is usually reserved for those in whom bleeding is likely to be severe. DDAVP may reduce blood loss in heavy bleeders but has been associated with increased risk of arterial thrombosis. Thromboelastography and other near-patient tests of haemostasis may be helpful in guiding treatment, although their value has not been rigorously established. For patients who need to continue taking aspirin until their operation, aprotinin may partially offset the anti-platelet effect.

Note: Recent reports suggest aprotinin may have previously unrecognised risks (page 15).

Liver transplantation and resection

Liver transplantation is confined to specialist centres familiar with the complex blood management problems that occur in these patients. Transfusion requirements have fallen greatly but substantial blood product support may still be needed because of preoperative coagulopathy due to liver disease, complex surgery with large blood losses and intra-operative coagulopathy with fibrinolysis that occurs during the anhepatic phase of the operation. Intra-operative blood salvage is important when there is major blood loss. Post-operatively, the risk of hepatic artery thrombosis may be reduced by avoiding over-transfusion with red cells and platelets. When a group O liver is transplanted to a group A or B patient, haemolytic anaemia may occur due to anti-A or anti-B antibodies produced in transplanted lymphoid tissue. Aprotinin is no longer used routinely, but at the discretion of the anaesthetist. Thromboelastography is commonly used as a guide to platelet and coagulation factor replacement.

Critical illness: anaemia and transfusion

Patients with critical illness often develop anaemia due to frequent blood sampling, gastrointestinal blood loss as a result of stress ulcers or gastric erosions, blood loss from intravascular lines and haemodialysis or haemofiltration circuits, impaired erythropoeitin production and direct marrow suppression by cytokines. Such patients often develop shock and multiple organ failure. Organ failure is probably partly due to an inadequate supply of oxygen to cells.

It is important to ensure sufficient oxygen supply to organs by maintaining adequate cardiac output, haemoglobin concentration, and haemoglobin saturation. These three factors determine the *oxygen delivery*. It used to be thought that survival could be improved by maintaining very high levels of oxygen delivery by transfusing red cells and giving drugs that increased cardiac output. This was called goal-directed therapy and a frequently used goal was a haemoglobin concentration > 100g/l.

It is now known that in most critically ill patients this level of haemoglobin concentration is not necessary. Most intensivists transfuse critically ill patients if their Hb falls below 80 g/l and maintain a concentration of 70–90 g/l. A possible exception to this guideline is for patients with known ischaemic heart disease. In this group many clinicians maintain a Hb > 90–100 g/l. ICU doctors no longer aim to achieve a predetermined oxygen delivery, but assess whether the oxygen delivery is adequate in individual patients by monitoring urine output, skin temperature, and the severity of lactic acidosis. Up to 50% of ICU admissions receive transfusion, and the ICU accounts for 5–6% of all red cells transfused.

Transfusion management: Critically ill patients often need transfusion because surgery or medical treatment is undertaken when the patient has a lowered Hb concentration and also a poor endogenous response to anaemia. Intravenous administration of iron may allow correction of Hb level in some cases (page 35).

Gastrointestinal haemorrhage: haematemesis and melaena (Tables 10 and 11)

- *Haematemesis*: vomiting fresh red blood.
- *Coffee-ground vomiting*: vomiting of altered black blood.
- *Melaena*: the passage of black tarry stools.
- Bleeding may be from *oesophageal varices* or from other sites (*non-variceal bleeding*).

Acute upper gastrointestinal (GI) bleeding affects 50 to 150 per 100,000 of the population each year and accounts for a substantial proportion of all blood used in UK hospitals. In the UK in 1995, mortality was reported to be 11% in patients admitted to hospital because of bleeding and 33% in those who developed gastrointestinal bleeding while hospitalised for other reasons. In the west of Scotland in 1997, the corresponding figures were 8.2% and 43%. Most deaths are in elderly patients with significant co-morbidity. Mortality is reported to be lower in specialist units where there is close medical/surgical/endoscopic cooperation and adherence to management protocols. This section is intended only to give an overview of transfusion, which is just one part of the overall management of patients with GI haemorrhage (Tables 10 and 11).

Transfusion management

Early recognition of significant blood loss is important. In clinical practice, it is commoner to see patients who have been under-transfused than over-transfused. It is essential to pay attention to and act on recordings of pulse rate and blood pressure. In a fit patient without cardiac disease, persistent tachycardia – even if blood pressure is maintained – is likely to indicate continuing blood loss.

All patients require *large-bore* intravenous cannulas. Central venous pressure monitoring is valuable in major haemorrhage or if there is cardio-respiratory disease.

Haemoglobin concentration – interpretation

The haemoglobin can underestimate the extent of blood loss in cases of acute haemorrhage before haemodilution has occurred, or can overestimate it if the patient is already anaemic from chronic blood loss.

If liver disease is suspected (e.g. oesophageal varices)

The platelet count and prothrombin time should be checked and correction with blood components may be indicated. It is not necessary to check clotting screen routinely in every case of GI haemorrhage.

Guidelines for management can be found at:
www.bsg.org.uk/clinical_prac/guidelines/nonvariceal.htm and
www.bsg.org.uk/clinical_prac/guidelines/man_variceal.htm

Table 10 Use of fluids and transfusion in GI bleeding in chronic liver disease (with variceal bleeding)

Features	Transfusion management	End points
Bleeding is often but not always from oesophageal varices and is often severe. Other causes such as peptic ulcer are not uncommon and must be excluded. Bleeding from varices usually recurs if there is no intervention to control the varices or to reduce portal pressure. The prognosis depends on the severity of the liver disease.* Hepatic failure may follow variceal bleeding, but usually recovers if bleeding can be stopped and recurrence prevented.[1]	Insert one or two large bore cannulas. A central line may be indicated. Ensure red cells are available quickly; use local emergency transfusion protocol: order 4–6 units. Crystalloids should be used carefully. Saline should be avoided as sodium retention is usual and leads to ascites.	Systolic pressure > 100 mmHg Urine output > 40 ml/hr CVP 0–5 mmHg (not higher) Haemoglobin up to 90 g/l
Thrombocytopenia is usual. Provided the platelet count is above 50×10^9/l, bleeding is unlikely to be controlled or prevented by platelet transfusion. Normal (i.e. pre-bleed) systolic blood pressure is often lower than in non-cirrhotic patients.	Platelet transfusion is rarely needed. If there is continued bleeding with a platelet count below 50×10^9/l, platelet transfusion may be considered in an effort to control variceal bleeding.	Platelet count may show little increment following platelet transfusion in patients with splenomegaly.
Deficiency of coagulation factors is frequent (except fibrinogen and factor VIII). Coagulation factor concentrates *may* be indicated. Seek expert advice as some of the products have a risk of thrombogenicity, especially in patients with liver disease.	Fresh frozen plasma is indicated only if there is documented coagulopathy, e.g. INR >2.0.	Keep INR < 2.0 if possible. Complete correction is rarely possible with FFP due to the large volume needed.
Giving red cells to try to raise Hb towards normal values may raise portal venous pressure, since blood volume is often increased. Over-transfusion may contribute to rebleeding. Provided blood volume is replaced and cardio-respiratory function was previously adequate, haemoglobin of 90 g/l appears to be adequate.	Transfuse red cells to approach but not exceed end point of 90 g/l.	

Note:

This table is based on the protocol used by the Gastrointestinal Bleeding Unit, Royal Infirmary, Aberdeen.
Masson J, Bramley PN, Herd K, McKnight GM, Park K, Brunt PW, McKinlay AW, Sinclair TS, Mowat NA, Upper gastrointestinal bleeding in an open-access dedicated unit, *J R Coll Physicians Lond*, 1996: 30(5):436–42.

Do:

- **group and save all patients**
- **act on vital signs**
- **use large-bore cannulas**
- **use CVP access in high risk patients**
- **correct coagulopathy in cirrhotics.**

Don't:

- **rely on Hb alone to guide red cell transfusion.**

Table 11 Use of fluids and blood components in acute non-variceal gastrointestinal bleeding

Severity	Clinical features	IV infusion	End point
Severe	History of collapse and/or shock – systolic BP < 100 mmHg – pulse > 100/min	Replace fluid rapidly Ensure red cells are available quickly; use local emergency transfusion protocol Transfuse red cells according to clinical assessment and Hb/Hct	Maintain urine output > 40 ml/hour systolic BP > 100 mmHg haemoglobin > 90 g/l
Significant	Resting pulse > 100/min and/or haemoglobin < 10 g/dl	Replacement fluid Order compatible red cells (four units)	Maintain haemoglobin > 90 g/l
Trivial	Pulse and haemoglobin normal	Maintain intravenous access until diagnosis is clear Send patient sample for red cell group and antibody screen	Recheck haemoglobin at 24 hours to reassess blood loss
No evidence of bleeding	May have 'coffee grounds' or altered blood in vomitus. Faecal occult blood negative.		

Note:

This table is based on the protocol used by the Gastrointestinal Bleeding Unit, Royal Infirmary, Aberdeen.

Masson J, Bramley PN, Herd K, McKnight GM, Park K, Brunt PW, McKinlay AW, Sinclair TS, Mowat NA, Upper gastrointestinal bleeding in an open-access dedicated unit, *J R Coll Physicians Lond*, 1996: 30(5):436–42.

Section 4
Clinical transfusion in the medical setting

Anaemia

Many patients who require transfusion have medical conditions and also undergo surgical interventions. Nevertheless, those who are seen in a 'medical' as opposed to a 'surgical' context have rather different causes of anaemia. A substantial proportion of patients receiving transfusion are elderly and have both 'medical' and 'surgical' features.

Features of patients seen in a medical or surgical context

Surgical	Medical
Acute blood loss	Chronic blood loss
Normal bone marrow	Bone marrow failure
Short term, recovering in short time	Long term, worsening without treatment
Transfusion threshold is the lowest physiologically acceptable Hb	Transfusion threshold takes account of fatigue, activity level, quality of life, ongoing therapy
Haematinic deficiency	Haematinic deficiency – nutrition or malabsorbtion
'Temporary anaemia of chronic disease' (see page 32)	Anaemia of chronic disease

Medical conditions and treatments likely to cause anaemia in patients in the UK are: solid tumours; haematological malignancies; peptic ulcer and other GI conditions; myelodysplasia; anaemia of chronic disease; poor nutrition; and treatment with chemotherapy and/or radiotherapy for malignant conditions. In many parts of the world, anaemia is very common mainly due to poor nutrition, malaria and parasite infestation.

Investigation and the plan of management should take account of possible causes, the severity of fatigue and other symptoms, the impact of co-morbidities, any likely effect of Hb level on outcome of therapy, the availability of specific treatment for the underlying disorder (e.g. steroids for autoimmune haemolytic anaemia, antilymphocyte globulin for aplastic anaemia, and chemotherapy for acute or chronic leukaemia) and the potential benefit of epoetin therapy.

Nutritional anaemias

Patients with iron, B12 and folate deficiency anaemias may present with a haemoglobin level below 50 g/l. Even these low levels are tolerated by some patients, and for these transfusion may be avoided since effective haematinic therapy will raise the Hb rapidly, reaching near normal in four to six weeks. Patients with severe anaemia due to vitamin B12 deficiency should be transfused with caution (a single unit, over three to four hours with close observation). It is not possible to recommend any single Hb value as a transfusion trigger in this group of patients. Each case should be treated on the basis of thorough clinical assessment. Transfusion will correct the anaemia but will not correct the deficiency state. This must be treated fully to prevent recurrence.

Treatment of iron deficiency

Oral iron
A standard regime is ferrous sulphate 200 mg tds (180mg elemental iron/day). Compliance with oral iron therapy is poor. Symptoms attributed to oral iron may be less if dose is reduced (e.g. 200 mg ferrous sulphate (65 mg of elemental iron) daily or 300 mg ferrous gluconate daily (35 mg of elemental iron)). If this is ineffective or not tolerated, parenteral iron may be considered.

Parenteral iron preparations
Indications: Severe iron deficiency anaemia with iron intolerance, malabsorption of oral iron or non-compliance with oral iron therapy. Patients with ongoing blood loss, anaemia of renal failure treated with epoetin.

Anaemia of chronic disease with EPO therapy, e.g. inflammatory bowel disease, rheumatoid arthritis.

Jehovah's Witnesses with iron deficiency and/or active blood loss.

Products: Two preparations are licensed in the UK: low molecular weight iron dextran (Cosmofer) and iron saccharate (Venofer).

Dosage and administration: Should be used according to manufacturer's directions and within local protocols.

Precautions

Immediate severe and potentially lethal anaphylactoid reactions can occur with parenteral iron-carbohydrate complexes. The risk is enhanced for patients with known (medical) allergy. When parenteral iron therapy is considered essential in patients with asthma, allergic disorders and inflammatory disorders, the intramuscular route is to be preferred.

CosmoFer® is an iron (III)-hydroxide dextran (low MW) complex. It may only be administered when anaphylactic emergency measures, including an injectable adrenaline solution, are available, i.e. adrenaline dose 0.5 ml of 1/1000 solution by intramuscular injection (**www.bnf.org**). Administration to patients with (auto)immune disorders or inflammatory conditions may cause a type III allergic reaction. Low MW iron dextran is associated with less adverse events than high MW dextran preparations.

Venofer® is an iron (III)-hydroxide sucrose complex. The most frequently reported adverse drug reactions (ADRs) in clinical trials were transient taste perversion, hypotension, fever and shivering, injection site reactions and nausea, occurring in 0.5 to 1.5% of the patients. Non-serious anaphylactoid reactions occurred rarely.

For dosage and administration, search **www.emc.medicines.org.uk**

Anaemia of chronic disease (ACD)

May contribute to anaemia in many situations where there is underlying malignancy, inflammation, sepsis and other conditions such as diabetes and congestive cardiac failure. The causes are a combination of: impaired marrow utilisation of iron; lower than expected rise in erythropoietin; blunted marrow response to erythropoietin; and erythroid activity suppressed by cytokines. These patients have an increased rate of transfusion as surgery or medical treatment commences with a lower haemoglobin level and with a poor endogenous response to anaemia. Intravenous administration of iron may allow correction of haemoglobin in some cases, and EPO therapy has also been successful, for instance, when used preoperatively in patients with rheumatoid arthritis awaiting joint replacement. Forward planning may reduce or eliminate the need for perioperative transfusion in some of these patients.

Anaemia in patients with cancer

Cancer may cause anaemia by infiltration of the bone marrow by cancer cells, impaired erythropoeisis due to inflammatory cytokines, nutritional deficiencies of iron and folate, blood loss into or from tumours, and kidney or liver damage, leading to reduced production of the hormone erythropoietin. Anti-cancer treatments, particularly platinum-containing drugs, can suppress the production of red blood cells in the bone marrow. Severe fatigue is perhaps the most commonly reported and debilitating symptom of anaemia in cancer. Other symptoms of anaemia, such as dizziness, shortness of breath on exertion, palpitations, headache and depression, also reduce the patient's quality of life. Many patients with cancer are anaemic at diagnosis. During treatment severity of anaemia fluctuates. It is typically worst two to four weeks after chemotherapy but depends on many factors, including the type of treatment and the number of courses. On completion of a course of treatment, haemoglobin tends to return to pre-treatment level, depending on how successful the treatment has been. In a large survey of patients with cancer, 39% had haemoglobin < 120 g/l at enrolment, 10% had haemoglobin < 100 g/l and 1% had haemoglobin < 80 g/l. More patients became anaemic during treatment.

The quality of life of patients with malignancy-associated anaemia may be improved by regular allogeneic red cell transfusion. Red cell transfusion is often a mainstay of supportive therapy in malignant conditions predominantly associated with marrow failure (such as myelodysplasia, myelofibrosis and aplastic anaemia) or extensive marrow infiltration (such as chronic lymphocytic leukaemia). Specific haematinic supplementation may be of benefit in any patient in whom vitamin deficiency has been identified. Iron therapy is often poorly tolerated.

Epoetin in anaemic cancer patients

Human erythropoietin is a glycoprotein hormone produced in the kidney. Epoetin is being used to prevent and treat anaemia in cancer patients. A recent Cochrane review found consistent evidence that the administration of epoetin reduces the risk for blood transfusions and the number of units transfused in anaemic cancer patients. However, it was not clear to what extent epoetin treatment affects quality of life or survival in such patients. A recent randomised trial of epoetin in patients with head and neck cancer showed poorer survival in the epoetin-treated patients, and a trial in breast cancer was halted when more tumour progression was observed in the epoetin arm of the trial. Some cancer cells express epoetin receptors, and epoetin may stimulate tumour blood vessel formation. A cautious approach to the use of epoetin in cancer patients is appropriate given the current state of knowledge. NICE has renewed epoetin for anaemia in cancer patients (**www.nice.org.uk**).

Licensed indications for epoetin products are given in the BNF. Epoetin should be used according to local hospital protocols.

Red cell transfusion

The patient's symptoms (fatigue, activity level) are the most important factor determining the need for transfusion. The ability to tolerate anaemia is affected particularly by respiratory function. The haemoglobin level is also usually monitored. If it is necessary to transfuse red cells to a patient with severe chronic anaemia, the risk of precipitating congestive cardiac failure may be minimised by ensuring the patient rests during the transfusion, administering a diuretic (e.g. frusemide 40–80 mg oral), and by reassessing the patient after the transfusion of each unit of red cells. The decision to give a diuretic must be based on clinical assessment of the patient: there are no clinical trials to provide guidance.

There are no clinical trials that compare the effect of maintaining Hb levels with epoetin versus red cell transfusion.

What haemoglobin concentration should be maintained?

It is felt by many clinicians that patients with conditions that lead to prolonged anaemia may need to be maintained with higher haemoglobin concentrations than patients experiencing surgery and critical illness. Studies in patients on dialysis for chronic renal failure indicate that there are benefits to patients' fatigue levels and other measures of quality of life if haemoglobin levels are maintained around 110 g/l.

Complications of long-term red cell transfusion

Special precautions are needed to avoid problems due to infection, alloimmunisation and iron overload in patients who need repeated transfusion of red cells over a long period. Before starting transfusions, patients should receive hepatitis B immunisation. Their red cell phenotype (at least Rh and Kell) should be determined and red cell units should be Rh and K matched to reduce risk of alloimmunisation. The routine use of leucocyte-depleted components in these patients reduces risk of adverse reactions due to white cell antibodies and cytokines in stored blood.

Iron overload: Patients with beta thalassaemia are the most likely to have iron overload problems, but patients with sickle cell disease and those with other transfusion-dependent conditions may also be affected. Each unit of red cells contains about 250 mg of iron. Since iron excretion is very limited, accumulation in the body causes toxic effects after 10–50 units have been transfused. These patients require life-long iron chelation therapy from the age of two to three years. Those who can comply well with iron chelation therapy have a 90% chance of surviving into the fourth decade of life; those who comply poorly have a high mortality rate in the third and fourth decade of life, usually due to complications of iron overload (cardiac disease, cirrhosis and diabetes mellitus).

Iron chelation therapy: A conventional regime would be desferioxamine 30–50 mg subcutaneously by slow infusion overnight using a syringe driver at least five times per week.

Haemoglobinopathies

All haemoglobins (Hb) consist of a *haem* (iron-containing) molecule bound to four globin chains (2 alpha and 2 non-alpha chains). The haem component is responsible for carrying oxygen, and the globin chains are essential for the stability, oxygen affinity and many other properties of the molecule. Inherited disorders of haemoglobin fall into two main categories. In the *thalassaemias* there is decreased or absent production of *normal* alpha or beta globin chains leading to reduced production of the main adult haemoglobin, Hb-A. These are very diverse disorders at the genetic and clinical levels. The *structural* Hb disorders result from mutations in the alpha or beta globin genes that alter the stability or function of the Hb molecule and are characterised by the presence of an abnormal Hb, such as sickle Hb (HbS). Haemoglobinopathies usually show autosomal recessive inheritance. Carriers of the abnormal gene (heterozygotes) are often asymptomatic, whereas those who inherit an abnormal gene from both parents (homozygotes) express the disease. Red cell transfusion is a common form of treatment in β-thalassaemia major and sickle-cell disease.

β-thalassaemia major

There are around 800 patients with this condition in the UK. Patients with this severe form of thalassaemia usually present with severe, life-threatening, anaemia before the age of one year as synthesis of fetal Hb (α and γ globin chains) switches to adult HbA (α and β, globin chains). They are then transfusion-dependent for life. The only cure for β-thalassaemia major is haemopoietic stem cell transplantation from a compatible donor. The cure rate is high in young children who have not yet developed severe iron overload from frequent red cell transfusions, but less than 30% of patients have an HLA-compatible family donor. Transplant-related mortality and morbidity is much higher in adults. Recently, the use of haemopoietic stem cells from the umbilical cord blood of HLA-compatible siblings or unrelated donors has shown very promising results. However, for the majority of patients, regular transfusions of red cells are the mainstay of treatment. Transfusions are given at two to four weekly intervals to maintain a mean Hb around 12 g/dl. The aim is to fully relieve the symptoms of anaemia and suppress the patient's own increased abnormal red cell production in the marrow (*ineffective erythropoiesis*) which causes the skeletal abnormalities and spleen enlargement seen in under-treated patients. All patients need *iron chelation* therapy (see above) to prevent progressive and ultimately fatal organ damage.

Sickle-cell disease

There are 12,000–15,000 individuals with sickle-cell disease in the UK. It is an autosomal recessive condition and only homozygotes have the full clinical picture (I IbSS) which is the most severe form. The sickle gene may also be found in combination with other abnormal haemoglobin genes common in the same populations, such as sickle-β-thalassaemia, which is variable in its severity, and SC disease (HbSC), which is usually milder. The characteristic features of all forms of sickle-cell disease are:

- chronic haemolytic anaemia
- recurrent acute sickle cell crises mainly affecting the long bones
- hyposplenism (due to splenic infarction) with an increased susceptibility to infection
- chronic organ damage due to recurrent sickling affecting particularly the CNS, liver, kidneys, bones/joints and lungs.

For most patients the mainstay of management is supportive with pain relief, fluids and antibiotics, and long-term folic acid supplements. Patients with severe disease causing stroke, acute chest syndrome or frequent painful sickling crises may be treated with hydroxyurea or, if age ≤ 16 years, allogeneic bone marrow transplantation from a related donor. Most patients require red cell transfusion intermittently and only to treat specific severe complications of the disease or in preparation for surgery.

The majority of patients with sickle-cell disease in the UK will receive red cell transfusion on several occasions during their life. Red cell transfusion is not usually indicated for acute sickle crisis, but exchange transfusion may be required for acute chest syndrome, intractable priapism, to prevent recurrence of stroke, for red cell aplasia (due to parvovirus infection) and to treat splenic or hepatic sequestration.

Exchange transfusion may be needed in acute stroke. The aim of exchange transfusion is to reduce the percentage of HbS to < 30% whilst keeping the haemoglobin below about 10 g/dl. In adults who have adequate venous access, exchange transfusion by cell separator may be performed by staff experienced in its use. Manual exchange transfusion is more often used for children. For major surgery and in some obstetric cases, prophylactic exchange transfusion is required. In aplastic or sequestration crises, top-up transfusion may be necessary.

Before transfusing any patient with sickle-cell disease, discuss with haematologist, as most patients are adapted to a Hb level around 6–8 g/dl, and raising the haemoglobin during an acute episode may worsen the crisis, causing microvascular damage.

Haemoglobinopathy trait

Patients who are carriers for haemoglobinopathies (thalassaemia or sickle-cell trait) are asymptomatic and never require transfusion on account of their haemoglobinopathy status.

Anaemia in chronic renal failure

Anaemia

Sixty to seventy per cent of patients with chronic renal failure (CRF) are anaemic. Many factors (iron deficiency, uraemia, hyperparathyroidism) contribute, but the principal cause is erythropoeitin deficiency. Epoetin is licensed for use in dialysis and pre-dialysis patients, and its use can almost eliminate the need for red cell transfusions. Many also have significant ischaemic heart disease, so perioperative anaemia should be avoided. A haemoglobin level of 100 g/l is commonly taken as a perioperative transfusion threshold for this group of patients. Epoetin is administered twice or thrice weekly. Epoetin-beta can be administered by intravenous or subcutaneous route. Epoetin-alpha can only be given intravenously. Parenteral iron saccharate can reduce the maintenance dose of epoetin.

Immunological sensitisation

Patients awaiting renal transplantation are exposed to particular risks by transfusion. Transfusion may stimulate broadly reactive antibodies against HLA class I antigens (allosensitisation) that increase the risk of renal allograft rejection and lead to poorer initial and long-term allograft survival. The principal risk factors for allosensitisation are the number of previous red cell transfusions, previous transplantation and previous pregnancy. Up to 30% of patients who have received 20 units of blood are allosensitised. Sustained high level of broadly reactive antibodies is mainly due to repeated transfusion. The switch to universal use of leucocyte-depleted blood in the UK will reduce the risk of HLA alloimmunisation. Several (but not all) studies show a decreased incidence of allosensitisation as well as a fall in antibody levels in sensitised patients. A guideline is available at **www.rcplondon.ac.uk/college/ceeu/amckd/index.asp**

Congenital haemostatic disorders

Patients with haemophilia A, haemophilia B (Christmas disease) and von Willebrand's disease

These patients should be registered with and cared for by a haemophilia centre. This centre should be contacted when a patient with haemophilia presents to another clinical unit. Many patients now receive recombinant factor VIII or factor IX products to minimise the risk of viral infection. Detailed guidance on the products recommended for management of these patients is published by the UK Haemophilia Centre Directors' Organisation (UKHCDO) and is regularly updated. When a patient with haemophilia is seen away from a specialist centre, it is important quickly to get the best help available. This is particularly important where a head injury is suspected, as treatment is often required urgently. For addresses of haemophilia centres in the UK, see **www.haemophilia.org.uk**

Initial care of a patient with haemophilia who has a bleed

- *Identification*: If the patient is unconscious, check if there is information carried on a bracelet or medallion.

- *Contact*: Contact the haemophilia centre for advice and inform the local haematologist. It is very important to ascertain the appropriate therapy and whether an inhibitor is known to be present. If the patient has suffered head injury, coagulation factor replacement should be started while these checks are being made.

- *Products for treatment*: Mild or moderate haemophilia A should be treated with DDAVP where possible. Patients with severe haemophilia A or B require factor VIII and IX concentrates respectively. The nearest supply may be in the patient's home. In general, treatment should be with the product that the patient normally uses. In a real emergency and if clotting factor concentrates are unavailable, cryoprecipitate is the appropriate treatment for severe haemophilia A and fresh frozen plasma that for haemophilia B.

- *Dosage*: Plasma-derived factor VIII in a dose of 1 iu/kg should give an immediate 2% rise in plasma factor VIII. Factor IX (1 iu/kg) should give an immediate 1% rise in factor IX level. Recombinant factor VIII requires a 30% higher dose for the same increment.

- *Monitoring*: Clotting factor levels are often needed to assess response to treatment. Contact the haematology department in your hospital or the haemophilia centre.

Von Willebrand's disease (vWD)

vWD is not straightforward to diagnose, and the assessment of a patient's treatment requirements or response to treatment can also be difficult. Measurements of the plasma levels of both factor VIII and von Willebrand factor are needed. For some procedures (and minor bleeding episodes) some patients can be managed with desmopressin (DDAVP) only. The patient's suitability for and response to DDAVP should be assessed by the haemophilia centre where the patient is first assessed. If clotting factor replacement is needed, a factor VIII concentrate must be chosen that contains vWF and is effective for vWD. Cryoprecipitate was formerly the chosen replacement therapy, but should only be used if a suitable virus-inactivated concentrate is not available.

Guidelines for management of patients with congenital coagulation disorders are available at **www.bcshguidelines.com**

Addresses for haemophilia treatment centres can be found at **www.haemophilia.org.uk/**

Bone marrow failure due to disease, cytotoxic therapy or irradiation

This section covers the use of platelet (Table 12) and red cell transfusion in situations where thrombocytopenia and anaemia commonly occur due both to the underlying disease and the effects of treatments including chemotherapy, radiation and antibiotics and antifungal drugs.

Table 12 Platelet transfusion in patients with bone marrow failure

Condition	Background	Threshold or target platelet count
Acute leukaemia	Clinical trials suggest that the threshold for prophylactic platelet transfusion in stable, uninfected patients can safely be lowered from 20×10^9/l.	Prophylactic platelet transfusion threshold 10×10^9/l.
Acute promyelocytic leukaemia	Coagulopathy may increase the risk of haemorrhage at any given platelet count.	Platelet count should be kept above 20×10^9/l if patient haemorrhagic.
Haemopoietic stem cell transplantation in acute leukaemia	Mucosal injury is more likely with transplantation than with chemotherapy alone, but studies indicate that the threshold for platelet transfusion can be lowered to 10×10^9/l. Duration of thrombocytopenia shorter with PBSC transplant than with BMT.	Prophylactic platelet transfusion threshold 10×10^9/l.
Chronic stable thrombocytopenia	Patients with chronic and sustained failure of platelet production (for example, some patients with myelodysplasia or aplastic anaemia) may remain free of serious haemorrhage, with platelet counts consistently below 10×10^9/l or even below 5×10^9/l. Long-term prophylactic platelet transfusions increase the risk of alloimmunisation with platelet refractoriness and other complications of transfusion.	In a patient who is otherwise stable, platelet transfusions should be restricted to treating haemorrhage. During unstable periods associated with infection or active treatment, prophylactic platelet transfusions may be needed to prevent recurrent bleeding.

Note on thresholds for platelet transfusion:

As a general guide, for this group of patients, a threshold platelet count of 10×10^9/l appears to be as safe as a higher level, for patients without additional risk factors. A threshold of 20×10^9/l should be observed in patients with risk factors such as sepsis, concurrent use of antibiotics or other abnormalities of haemostasis.

Patients with chronic stable thrombocytopenia are best managed on an individual basis depending on the degree of haemorrhage.

Patients with chronic stable thrombocytopenia are best managed on an individual basis depending on the degree of haemorrhage.

ABO and RhD compatibility of platelet transfusions
ABO incompatibility can reduce the expected platelet count increment (CI) by 10–30%.

If it is necessary to give RhD positive cellular blood components to a female with childbearing potential, anti RhD immunoglobulin should be given to avoid the risk of the patient developing RhD antibodies (see page 52). The dose of anti RhD immunoglobulin is 125 iµ per ml of red cells transfused.

Platelet refractoriness
Refractoriness is defined as a repeated failure to achieve a satisfactory increment after two or more platelet transfusions. The platelet count the morning after transfusion should be raised by at least 20×10^9/l. If the increase is persistently less than 20×10^9/l this suggests refractoriness. Non-immune causes include infection, fever, splenomegaly, DIC and treatment with antifungals such as amphotericin or antibiotics such as ciprofloxacin. Immune causes are anti-HLA or anti-platelet antibodies, e.g. anti-HPA1a.

Management of refractoriness
It is important to identify refractoriness due to HLA or antiplatelet antibodies as compatible platelet transfusions may be more effective. Poor responses to HLA-matched platelets could also be due to ABO antibodies or to unrecognised non-immune causes. Further guidance on diagnosis and management is available in British Committee for Standards in Haematology (BCSH) guidelines.

Red cell transfusion

The local clinical management protocol should define the range within which a patient's haemoglobin should be maintained. A suggested arbitrary guide is to maintain Hb at not less than 9.0 g/dl.

Prevention of transfusion-associated graft-versus-host disease (TA-GvHD)

Transfused donor lymphocytes which are compatible with the recipient, but which recognise the recipient as foreign, can engraft and initiate TA-GvHD. Patients develop skin rash, diarrhoea and abnormal liver function, and deteriorate, with bone marrow failure and death from infection usually within two to three weeks of transfusion. TA-GvHD can be prevented by gamma irradiating (25 Gy dose) the blood components to be transfused. This inactivates the donor lymphocytes. Leucocyte depletion cannot be considered to remove risk of TA-GvHD. Patients requiring irradiated blood should be given an information leaflet and card available from blood centres, informing them about their need for irradiated blood and the fact that they should make clinical staff aware of this. (see page 42).

Prevention of cytomegalovirus transmission (Table 14)

Cytomegalovirus (CMV) infection can cause serious morbidity in immunocompromised CMV-negative patients. The risk can be minimised by the use of CMV-antibody-negative (seronegative) blood components. Leucocyte depletion also confers some protection since the virus is associated with white blood cells. A consensus conference in 2001 concluded that components that are both CMV-seronegative and leucodepleted should be used for CMV-seronegative pregnant women, intrauterine transfusions, and CMV-seronegative-allogeneic stem cell transplant recipients. Some studies, however, suggest that effective leucodepletion may confer as much protection as the use of CMV-negative components.

Table 13 Transfusion support in stem cell transplant patients with donor/recipient ABO incompatibility

In a patient who has received an ABO-incompatible stem cell transplant, the transplant may express a new A and/or B antigen from the donor (major mismatch) or a new A and/or B antibody from the donor (minor mismatch)

Blood components for transfusion should be according to the following guidance

	Red cells	Plasma and platelets
Major ABO mismatch	Use red cells of the recipient's ABO type until recipient ABO antibodies are undetectable and the DAT is negative	*Use plasma (and platelets) of the recipient's ABO type*
Minor ABO mismatch	Use red cells of the donor ABO type throughout	Use plasma and platelets of the recipient type until recipient-type red cells are no longer detectable
Major plus minor ABO mismatch	*Use group O red cells until recipient ABO antibodies are undetectable and then change to red cells of the donor's type*	Use group AB plasma and platelets until recipient-type red cells are undetectable

Table 14 Indications for the use of CMV-antibody-negative and gamma-irradiated cellular blood components[1]

CMV-antibody-negative components

CMV-antibody-negative pregnant women

CMV-antibody-negative recipients of allogeneic stem cell grafts

Intrauterine transfusions (IUT)

Patients with HIV disease

Gamma-irradiated components

Transfusions from first- or second-degree relatives

Any granulocyte transfusion for any recipient

HLA-selected platelet units

Patients receiving purine analogues (fludarabine, cladribine, deoxycoformycin): probably safer to use indefinitely

Intrauterine transfusion (IUT)

Exchange transfusion (provided that irradiation does not unduly delay transfusion)

Red cell or platelet transfusion in neonates – only if there has been a previous IUT or if blood is from first- or second-degree relative

All recipients of allogeneic haemopoietic stem cell (HSC) grafts, from start of conditioning therapy and while patient remains on GvHD prophylaxis

Blood transfused to allogeneic HSC donors before or during the harvest of their HSC

Patients who will have autologous HSC graft:
- any transfusion within 7 days of the collection of their HSC
- any transfusion from the start of conditioning therapy until:
  ○ 3 months post transplant
  ○ 6 months post transplant if conditioning TBI has been given

Hodgkin's disease, at all stages of the disease

Congenital immunodeficiency with defective cell-mediated immunity (e.g. SCID, Di George syndrome, Wiskott Aldrich syndrome, purine nucleoside deficiency, reticular dysgenesis, ADA, Ataxia telangectasia, chronic mucosal candidiasis, MHC class 1 or 2 deficiency)

Notes:
[1] Red cells, platelets and granulocyte components must be irradiated for all at-risk patients. It is not necessary to irradiate fresh frozen plasma, cryoprecipitate, cryosupernatant or plasma derivatives.

[2] It is not necessary to irradiate components for patients with solid tumours, organ transplants, HIV or aplastic anaemia.

[3] As new cytotoxic and immunosuppressive agents, including monoclonal antibodies, are introduced, these guidelines will be updated.

Immunological disorders – use of immunoglobulin (Table 15)

Human normal immunoglobulin products are derivatives of pooled normal donor plasma. They are used as long-term replacement therapy for missing or defective immunoglobulin in patients with antibody deficiency disorders and also, in much higher doses (usually in short courses), as immunomodulatory agents in patients with a range of autoimmune or inflammatory conditions.

Hyperimmune immunoglobulins are prepared from donors selected for possession of particular antibody specificities and are used for passive immunisation against specific infections or to avoid potentially harmful immune reactions. One such product, anti RhD immunoglobulin, is used to inhibit the immune response to the RhD antigen (see page 52).

Primary antibody deficiency (primary hypogammaglobulinaemia)

The term primary antibody deficiency (PAD) encompasses a range of inherited disorders characterised by defects in antibody production and/or function. Specialist advice on diagnosis and management should be sought as these patients require detailed assessment for selection and adjustment of treatment regimens. They also need to be monitored for acute and chronic complications of both disease and treatments and to assess the efficacy of treatment. Immunoglobulin replacement therapy should only be instituted for patients meeting defined diagnostic criteria for PAD or where there is strong suspicion that some other, indefinable antibody deficiency disorder is present. Immunoglobulin replacement is the mainstay of treatment for PAD.

Intravenous immunoglobulin (IVIgG) is formulated for intravenous administration and is usually given by infusion every three to four weeks. Subcutaneous immunoglobulin (SCIgG) is formulated differently to IVIgG and is given by weekly, pump-delivered subcutaneous infusion. SCIgG should never be given intravenously. Dose and frequency of administration of IVIgG or SCIgG should be adjusted to maintain serum IgG levels above a minimum of 5 g/l. In children with some types of

PAD syndromes (e.g. x-linked agammaglobulinaemia) a higher level – above 8 g/l – may prevent chronic disease complications. Complications, such as chronic lung damage or mycoplasma arthritis, may also be indications to maintain higher IgG levels.

Intramuscular immunoglobulin (IMIgG) is no longer recommended for treatment of patients with PAD. The weekly injections required are painful, adequate IgG levels cannot be achieved or maintained, and adverse reactions are common. IMIgG should never be given by the intravenous route.

Guidelines are available at **www.ukpin.org.uk/**

Secondary antibody deficiency

Defects of antibody production and/or function can occur in a variety of neoplastic, inflammatory infectious (including HIV), metabolic, traumatic, nutritional and drug-induced disorders. In many cases the antibody deficiency is minor and is corrected by effective management of the primary, underlying disorder. In some situations (e.g. in some patients with chronic lymphatic leukaemia or myeloma), antibody replacement therapy may be indicated and should be managed along the same lines as PAD.

Dosage and administration of IVIgG and SCIgG in primary or secondary antibody deficiency

Prior to commencement of immunoglobulin replacement therapy: The clinician responsible should assess the risks and benefits of immunoglobulin therapy for the individual patient. The patient should receive written information about his/her condition and the treatment options, and should give written, informed consent to the treatment. Pre-treatment liver function tests and a hepatitis RNA test should be done and a serum sample archived.

Dose: For most patients either IV infusion of 200–600 mg/kg every three to four weeks or sub-cutaneous infusion of 100–150 mg/kg weekly is appropriate. Infusion rates in the product information instructions must be followed, both at the start of treatment and during subsequent infusions. Incorrect infusion rate is a common cause of adverse reactions. Dosing and frequency of infusions should be adjusted according to symptoms and the results of monitoring so as to maintain serum IgG above minimum of 5 g/l. Batch numbers of all immunoglobulin products used should be recorded and retained indefinitely along with date(s) of administration.

Precautions: It is essential to adhere to the infusion rates specified in the package insert. These are designed to minimise the risk of acute reactions. The daily maximum dose of 1 g/kg must not be exceeded on any one day. The maximum dose of 2 g/kg must not be exceeded in any single course of treatment. In elderly patients a daily dose of 0.4 g/kg daily over five days may be a safer way of administering the course of treatment.

Monitoring of treatment: Regular weighing of the patient will help guide immunoglobulin dosage requirements and is particularly important in children. Laboratory tests should include regular liver function tests, C-reactive protein, and pre-infusion serum immunoglobulin levels. Patients should have an annual test for hepatitis C RNA. Serum samples should be archived on a regular basis. Batch numbers of all immunoglobulin products administered must be recorded.

Immunomodulatory therapy with high-dose intravenous immunoglobulin

High doses of IVIgG have shown benefit in many conditions, and the indications have broadened over the past 10 years. The mechanism(s) of action include blocking Fc receptors, anti-inflammatory effects and effects on T and B lymphocytes. IVIgG infusion can cause severe adverse reactions. Because the product is expensive and often in short supply, it should only be prescribed for conditions where there is good evidence of its effectiveness.

Indications: Indications are summarised in Table 15.

Adverse events associated with high-dose IVIgG

Renal failure has occurred following administration of high doses of IVIgG, usually in elderly patients. Predisposing factors are pre-existing renal impairment, diabetes and paraproteinaemia. Rapid infusion increases the risk of anaphylactoid and other acute reactions. These reactions are at least in part due to the stabilisers used in formulating the products. Patients who react to one manufacturer's product may tolerate a different formulation.

Therapeutic plasma exchange (Table 16)

Therapeutic plasma exchange (TPE) involves extra-corporeal processing of a patient's blood to remove large-molecular-weight substances from the plasma. Such substances are pathogenic auto-antibodies (e.g. Myasthenia Gravis: autoantibody to acetyl cholinesterase receptor), cryoglobulins or other abnormal plasma proteins (e.g. Waldenstrom's macroglobulinaemia: monoclonal immunoglobulin) or immune complexes (e.g. Goodpasture's syndrome: autoantibody to basement membrane). Several treatments are usually given. Typically 30–40 ml/kg of plasma (1–1.5 plasma volumes) are removed and replaced with albumin or albumin and normal saline during each procedure. The procedure must be controlled to ensure that the patient is kept in fluid balance, maintaining a stable, normal plasma volume. A single exchange removes approximately 75% of the patient's own

Table 15 Conditions where IVIgG may have benefit

Speciality	Condition	Prerequisites for consideration of IVIgG treatment	Dosing schedule	Monitoring
Immunology	Primary immunodeficiency	Hypogammaglobulinaemia deficient total IgG or subclass deficiency	0.2 g/kg 3–4 weekly	Titre dose against levels and bacterial infections
Haematology	Idiopathic thrombocytopenic purpura + HIV-associated ITP	Life threatening haemorrhage or rapid increase in platelet count required or steroid contraindicated	1 g/kg with second dose at 24 hours dependent on response	Platelet count
	Allogeneic BMT for prevention of GvHD	Allogeneic BMT	0.5 g/kg day weekly to d+90	
	NAITP	Affected pregnancy with homozygous father or fetal platelet count $< 100 \times 10^9/l$	1 g/kg/week from 20/40 weeks	Fetal platelet count
	PTP	Severely affected patient	1 g/kg/day × 2 days	Platelet count
	Secondary hypogammaglobulinaemia	CLL/myeloma with low IgG levels and > 2 bacterial infections in 12-month period	0.2 g/kg monthly	Reduction in infections
Neurology	GBS + Miller Fisher syndrome	Severe disease where TPE not immediately available	0.4 g/kg/day × 5 days	May be repeated if some measure of response
	CIDP + multifocal motorneuropathy	Steroid treatment failed, not appropriate, or steroid side effects anticipated	0.4 g/kg/day × 5 days, then 1 g/kg 4–6 weekly	Stop once plateau achieved
	Myasthenia gravis + LEMS	Acute exacerbations where TPE unavailable	1 g/kg/day × 2 days	
	Acute disseminated encephalomyelitis	Failed high dose steroids	1 g/kg/day × 2 days	
Rheumatology	DM + PM	Active recalcitrant disease which has failed immunosuppression	1 g/kg/day × 2 days	Repeated doses may be required
	SLE	Only where thrombocytopenia is the major complication	1 g/kg/day × 2 days	Platelet count
	Kawasaki's disease		1–2 g/kg over 2–5 days	
Dermatology	Pemphigus Vulgaris/ Bullous Pemphigoid	Recalcitrant disease as an adjuvant to immunosuppressants	1 g/kg × 2–5 days given monthly	Stop once lesions healed
	Toxic epidermal necrolysis		1–2 g/kg over 2–5 days	
	Chronic urticaria	Failed conventional therapy	1–2 g/kg over 2–5 days	Stop after 3 courses
Infectious diseases	Neonatal sepsis		1–2 g/kg over 2–5 days	
	Toxic shock/ necrotising fasciitis	Adjuvant treatment to antibiotics and supportive care	1 g/kg × 1 day, then 0.5 g/kg × 2 days	

plasma and the abnormal constituent in the plasma. A series of three consecutive daily plasma exchanges will remove about 95% of a circulating IgG antibody. Thrombotic thrombocytopenia (TTP) is treated by plasma exchange with FFP (page 45) to replace VWF cleaving enzyme and remove antibody.

Clinical indications for therapeutic plasma exchange (Table 16)

It is advised that PE should normally only be considered in conditions where well-designed clinical trials or a broad base of published experience support its use. These are thrombotic thrombocytopenic purpura (TTP), Guillain-Barré syndrome, chronic inflammatory demyelinating polyneuropathy (CIDP), and renal disease with antiglomerular basement membrane antibody. Other conditions in

Table 16 Therapeutic plasma exchange: indications

Speciality	Condition
Neurology	Acute Guillain-Barré syndrome
	Chronic inflammatory demyelinating polyneuropathy
	Myasthenia gravis
Haematology	Hyperviscosity syndromes
	Thrombotic thrombocytopenic purpura (exchange with plasma)
	Cryoglobulinaemias
	Post-transfusion purpura
Renal	Goodpasture's syndrome
	ANCA (antineutrophil cytoplasmic antigen) positive nephritis
Metabolic	Refsum's disease
	Hypercholesterolaemia

which PE is generally accepted as having a supportive role are rapidly progressive glomerulone-phritis, cryoglobulinaemia, myeloma with paraproteins and hyperviscosity and Lambert-Eaton myasthenic syndrome. In TTP, TPE must be performed with plasma as this is more effective than simple plasma infusion. For all the other conditions mentioned, TPE is performed with albumin or saline.

Thrombotic thrombocytopenic purpura
The Department of Health policy is now to use solvent-detergent FFP (SDFFP) for thrombotic thrombocytopenic purpura (TTP). Precautions against thromboembolism are recommended (graduated elastic compression stockings at diagnosis and prophylactic low-molecular-weight heparin once the platelet count rises above $50 \times 10^9/l$).

Risks of TPE

Bruises or haematomas at venepuncture site. Inadequate vascular access can compromise the procedure due to low flow or thrombosis. Effects of citrate anticoagulant, such as perioral tingling, parasthesia (due to low ionised calcium). Urticaria or anaphylaxis or haemolysis due to plasma infusion, fluid overload or under-replacement, vasovagal attack.

Haemostatic changes
PT and APTT are mildly prolonged immediately after plasma exchange due to removal and dilution of plasma proteins, but show substantial recovery within 4 to 24 hours. About 10 to 15% of the platelets are lost during each exchange. The levels of fibrinogen and other coagulation factors fall considerably by the end of the procedure: this leads to prolonged blood clotting tests, although a clinically significant bleeding tendency does not usually result. Fibrinogen and coagulation screen should be checked after the procedure, especially if any surgical intervention or biopsy is to be performed.

Apheresis to remove other abnormal blood constituents

Red cells: Abnormal red cells are removed and replaced with normal red cell components. See page 38 for sickle-cell disease.

White cells: Patients with very high white cell counts ($> 300 \times 10^9/l$) in chronic myeloid leukaemia may have signs and symptoms due to leucostasis. Reduction of the white count by removal of leucocytes may benefit the patient until definitive chemotherapy takes effect.

Lymphocytes: Photopheresis employs apheresis to separate T cells from the blood so that they can be exposed to UV irradiation and a photosensitising agent and then re-infused. This procedure is used in patients with cutaneous T cell lymphoma.

Immunoadsorption

Plasma is removed by means of an apheresis device, passed over an adsorption medium to remove a specific constituent and returned to the patient. Adsorbents used include Staphylococcal Protein A (binds the Fc portion of IgG molecules), immobilised antibodies and dextran. Applications include removal of antibodies to factor VIII in acquired haemophilia and reduction of plasma lipids in familial hyperlipidaemia.

A recent guideline, based on a systematic review of the literature, is available at
www.apheresis.org/

Section 5
Immunoglobulin for prevention of infection (Table 17)

Whenever possible, patients should be vaccinated against infections rather than be given immunoglobulins. In some situations human normal immunoglobulin (HNIG) or specific immunoglobulins for varicella-zoster, hepatitis B, rabies and tetanus may be used, often together with active immunisation, to protect against infection. Supplies of immunoglobulins and practical clinical information about their use can be obtained from the Health Protection Agency's Centre for Infections (020 8200 4400) or from blood transfusion centres in Scotland.

Dosage, precautions, contraindications and side effects: Refer to Table 17 and individual product information. Further information can be found at:
www.hpa.org.uk/infections/topics_az/immunoglobulin/menu.htm

Table 17 Immunoglobulins for prevention of infection

For more information go to **www.hpa.org.uk/infections/topics_az/immunoglobulin/4.pdf**

Infection	Indications	Preparations, vial content	Dose (by intramuscular injection)
Hepatitis A	Household and other close contacts Outbreaks where there is a clearly defined exposure if there has been delay in identifying cases	Human normal immunoglobulin (HNIG) 250 mg and 750 mg	< 10 years 250 mg ≥ 10 years 500 mg
Tetanus	High-risk wounds in immunised individuals or any tetanus-prone wound in incompletely immunised or unimmunised individuals	Human tetanus immunoglobulin (HTIG) 250 iu	250 iu (500 iu if > 24 hours since injury, risk of heavy contamination, or following burns)
Measles	Immunosuppressed contacts, pregnant women, infants < 10 months	Human normal immunoglobulin (I INIG) 250 mg and 750 mg	250 mg < 1 year 500 mg 1–2 years 750 mg ≥ 3 years
Rubella	Pregnant women only	Human normal immunoglobulin (HNIG) 750 mg	750 mg
Mumps	Not recommended	–	–
Polio	Immunosuppressed persons, or contacts of, inadvertently given live polio vaccine	Human normal immunoglobulin (HNIG) 750 mg	250 mg < 1 year 500 mg 1–2 years 750 mg ≥ 3 years
Hepatitis B	Accidental exposure, including needlestick, or mucosal/non-intact skin exposure Sexual exposure	Human hepatitis B immunoglobulin (HBIG) 200 iu or 500 iu	200 iu 0–4 years 300 iu 5–9 years 500 iu ≥ 10 years
Hepatitis B	Newborn babies of high-risk mothers	Hepatitis B immunoglobulin (HBIG) 100 iu	200 iu
Chickenpox	Immunosuppressed patients, pregnant women and neonates who are significantly exposed to chickenpox or herpes zoster and have no antibodies to varicella-zoster virus	Varicella-zoster immunoglobulin (VZIG) 250 mg and 500 mg vials	250 mg 0–5 years 500 mg 6–10 years 750 mg 11–14 years 1000 mg ≥ 15 years Give second dose if further exposure and 3 weeks have lapsed since first dose.
Rabies	Bite or mucous membrane exposure to potentially rabid animals or an animal unavailable for observation	Human rabies immunoglobulin (HRIG) 500 iu	20 iu/kg
Sources of supply	The following preparations for intramuscular use are issued by Immunisation Department of HPA Communicable Disease Surveillance Centre (020 8327 7773) and certain local Health Protection Agency and NHS public health laboratories: • human normal immunoglobulin (HNIG) • human varicella-zoster immunoglobulin (VZIG) • human hepatitis B immunoglobulin (HBIG) • human rabies immunoglobulin (HRIG). Or contact your local pharmacy or blood transfusion centre.		

Comments

Vaccine is preferred to HNIG, except if there has been delay of one week or more in identifying cases and/or an individual is at high risk of severe disease because of coexisting liver disease or patient is immunosuppressed, or the outbreak is in a population likely to experience morbidity. HNIG is no longer recommended for travel prophylaxis.

Administer **with a full course of combined tetanus/low dose diphtheria vaccine (Td)**
in the following:
(i) unimmunised/incompletely immunised subjects
(ii) immunisation history unknown/uncertain.

HNIG is most effective if given within 72 hours, but can be effective even if given within 6 days. Immunocompromised patients should be given HNIG as soon as possible. Infants from 9 months should be given MMR vaccine. HNIG may not be required for infants < 6 months as they are likely to have maternal antibody.
Seek further advice from HPA.

HNIG should be used when termination is not acceptable to a non-immune pregnant woman. HNIG does not prevent infection, but may reduce the likelihood of clinical symptoms. Neither MMR nor rubella vaccine are effective for post-exposure prophylaxis.

HNIG and MMR vaccine are not effective for post-exposure protection, and there is no mumps-specific immunoglobulin.

HNIG should be given as soon as possible after exposure. History of prior vaccination should be taken and serum for antibody determination obtained.

Administer **with hepatitis B vaccine** preferably within 12 hours and not later than 1 week after exposure. Individuals who have been successfully vaccinated (≥ 10mIU/ml 3 months after the third dose) require a booster dose of vaccine ONLY, unless booster given in the past year. Vaccine non-responders (< 10 iu) should be given a second dose of HBIG 1 month after the first unless the source is shown to be HBsAg negative.

Administer **with hepatitis B vaccine** as soon as possible and within 48 hours to babies born to mothers who either had acute hepatitis B in pregnancy, or are persistent carriers of HBsAg, where HBsAg is detectable or anti HBe is not.

Immunosuppressed patients are defined as:
(i) undergoing (or within 6 months of) chemotherapy or generalised radiotherapy; (ii) organ recipients on immunosuppressive treatment; (iii) bone marrow recipients, who are considered to be immunosuprressed; (iv) patients on (or within 3 months of) daily high-dose steroids for more than a week (e.g. children: 2 mg/kg/day, adults: 40 mg/kg/day of prednisolone); (v) patients on lower dose steroids, given in combination with cytotoxic drugs; (vi) patients with evidence of impaired cell-mediated immunity; (vii) symptomatic HIV-positive patients or asymptomatic with low CD4+ counts.
Patients with gammaglobulin deficiencies who are receiving replacement therapy with IV HNIG *do not require* VZIG.

Pregnant women: VZ-antibody-negative pregnant contacts at any stage of pregnancy, providing VZIG can be given < 10 days of contact (count days from onset of rash for household contacts). Pregnant contacts with a positive history do not require VZIG; those with a negative history must be tested for VZ antibody before VZIG is given.

Neonates: (i) VZIG should be given to infants whose mothers develop chickenpox (but not zoster) in the period 7 days before to 7 days after delivery, with or without antibody testing. It should also be given to VZ-antibody-negative infants (based on antenatal/infant blood sample) exposed to chickenpox or zoster in first 7 days of life. (ii) Infants who are premature, low birth weight or on SCBU: VZIG should be given to infants born < 28 weeks, weighing < 1 kg and had repeated blood sampling, or > 60 days old and exposed to chickenpox or herpes zoster.

Administer **with rabies vaccine** according to country risk and immunisation status. See HPA rabies protocol available at:
www.hpa.org.uk/infections/topics_az/rabies/hpa_Rabies_protocol_August_2003.pdf

Section 6
Transfusion in antenatal obstetric and neonatal care

Obstetric haemorrhage (Figures 1a and 1b, Table 18)

There were 17 maternal deaths directly due to haemorrhage reported to the UK Confidential Enquiry during 2000–2002. The obstetric conditions were: placenta praevia, placental abruption and postpartum haemorrhage (10 cases of PPH, compared to a single case in the previous three-year period). Five further deaths involved complications in which significant haemorrhage occurred (eclampsia, placenta accreta at termination of pregnancy, amniotic fluid embolism and ruptured uterus). For more information search **www.cemach.org.uk**.

The blood flow to the placenta is about 700 ml/min at term, so bleeding is likely to be rapid. It is often unexpected and difficult to control. Disseminated intravascular coagulation is common in obstetric haemorrhage due to placental abruption, amniotic fluid embolism and intrauterine death. Haemorrhage due to obstetric DIC is usually relieved only by treating the underlying disorder. Supportive treatment with platelets, FFP and cryoprecipitate may be required and should be guided by laboratory tests. Bleeding into the uterine cavity, the uterine wall or the abdomen may conceal the extent of the blood loss. As a result, the patient may decompensate suddenly in the post-delivery period.

Table 18 Successful transfusion management of obstetric haemorrhage – key factors

See major haemorrhage protocol, Figures 1a and 1b.

Use of a comprehensive management protocol with which all staff are familiar.

Clear communication between the hospital transfusion laboratory and the labour ward (see major haemorrhage protocol, inside front cover).

An agreed code or form of words that will:

- alert blood bank staff to the need for urgent delivery of group O RhD negative blood (or blood of the patient's own ABO and Rh group)

- avoid life-threatening delay due to performance of a full crossmatch. This is inappropriate when there is life-threatening bleeding.

Regular 'fire drills' to familiarise all staff and to test the success of the protocol.

Training and competence assessment of the staff who transport samples and blood.

Rapid and effective transfusion and haematology lab support.

Reliable availability at the blood bank of uncrossmatched, group-compatible blood within 10–15 minutes of receipt of a blood sample.

A standing agreement between the haematologists and obstetricians over the issue of platelets, FFP and/or cryoprecipitate, which reduces the number of phone calls required and speeds response.

Agreement that initial transfusion of blood components does not require to await results of coagulation tests (see major haemorrhage protocol, inside front cover).

Rapidly available coagulation monitoring results, which will help to assess the adequacy of the coagulation support and guide the selection of components.

Availability of intra-operative cell salvage for:

- Jehovah's Witness patients, and

- patients with placenta praevia accreta.

Haemolytic disease of the newborn

Pregnancies potentially affected by HDN should be cared for by specialist teams with facilities for early diagnosis, intrauterine transfusion and support of high-dependency neonates.

Haemolytic disease of the newborn (HDN) occurs when the mother has anti-red-cell IgG antibodies in her plasma that cross the placenta and bind to fetal red cells bearing the corresponding antigen. The three most common red cell alloantibodies which cause significant HDN are anti D, anti c and anti Kell (anti K). Fetal red cells binding sufficient maternally derived antibody are destroyed in the fetal reticuloendothelial system, producing extravascular haemolysis and a variable degree of fetal anaemia. In severe cases the fetus may die *in utero* of heart failure (*hydrops fetalis*). If the fetus survives birth, the neonate rapidly develops jaundice and is at risk of neurological damage due to the high bilirubin level.

Development of red cell antibodies in the mother may occur either as a result of previous pregnancies (because fetal blood displaying paternal red cell antigens frequently enters the mother's circulation during pregnancy) or as a result of a previous blood transfusion.

The most important cause of HDN is antibody to the RhD antigen (anti D). This develops in RhD negative women who have carried a RhD positive fetus. It rarely affects the first pregnancy although it can sensitise the mother so that subsequent pregnancies with RhD positive babies boost antibody production progressively, putting later pregnancies at increasing risk. Smaller family sizes and the introduction of prophylaxis with RhD immunoglobulin have reduced the incidence and severity of this condition.

The fetus is only at risk if its red blood cells express the antigens against which the antibody is directed (e.g. if a RhD negative woman with anti D is carrying a RhD positive fetus, there is a risk that the fetus will be affected, but if the fetus is RhD negative the baby will not be at risk of HDN).

The next most common causes of severe HDN are the rhesus antibody anti c or Kell antibody (anti K). In HDN due to anti K, the antibody also causes reduced fetal red cell production. This is due to anti K binding to red cell progenitor cells; in such cases the anaemia is often very severe while jaundice may be minimal.

Although it is not usually severe, the most common form of HDN is that caused by antibodies of the ABO blood group system in a group O mother with naturally occurring anti-A and anti-B of the IgG subclass which can cross the placenta. HDN due to ABO incompatibility occurs when a group O mother with IgG anti-A or IgG anti-B is carrying a fetus of blood group A or blood group B respectively. The most common presentation of ABO HDN is jaundice (unconjugated hyperbilirubinaemia). The direct antiglobulin test is usually (but not always) positive. Severe anaemia in HDN due to maternal anti-A or anti-B is uncommon in Caucasians in the UK, but is commoner in some other ethnic groups, especially among women of African or Caribbean origin.

Prevention of HDN due to anti RhD (Table 19)

Refer to BCSH 2006 Guideline at www.bcshguidelines.com

Anti RhD immunoglobulin (anti D)

Anti-D immunoglobulin is prepared from plasma of donors who have high levels of plasma anti-D due to exposure to RhD positive cells following pregnancy or intentional immunisation. Anti-D products contain specified levels of anti D and are available for intramuscular or intravenous administration. Anti D is administered to RhD negative women who may have been exposed to RhD positive fetal red cells that have entered the maternal circulation. The anti D destroys the RhD positive red cells and prevents active immunisation, thus preventing the production of RhD antibodies.

Potentially sensitising events during pregnancy

Potentially sensitising events (PSEs) are events that may cause feto-maternal bleeding (Table 19) and can cause the mother to develop anti D. If the pregnancy has reached 20 weeks or longer, patients with any of these events should receive anti D followed by a test that determines the volume of fetal red cells in the maternal circulation (a Kleihauer test or equivalent), as it may be necessary to give a bigger dose of anti D if more than 4 ml of fetal cells entered the mother's circulation. An additional 125 iu/ml of red cells will be required. If there is repeated antepartum haemorrhage (APH) during the pregnancy, further doses of anti D should be given at six-weekly intervals. Patients with potentially sensitising events may present to hospital accident and emergency departments or to their general practitioner. It is important that these staff are aware of the risks of sensitisation so that patients can receive anti D when it is indicated.

Routine antenatal anti-D prophylaxis

The National Institute for Clinical Excellence has recommended that routine antenatal anti-D prophylaxis (RAADP) be offered to all non-sensitised pregnant women who are RhD negative at 28 and 34 weeks of pregnancy. This is to reduce the residual number of mothers at risk (about 1.5%) who still develop anti D from pregnancies. Potentially sensitising events occurring around the time of RAADP still require to be managed with additional doses of anti D and Kleihauer (or equivalent) testing. See www.nice.org.uk

See notes on alternative dose regimes in Table 19.

Table 19 Prophylaxis of Rh haemolytic disease of the newborn

Screening for HDN in pregnancy (see BCSH Guideline: blood grouping and antibody testing during pregnancy)

- At the time of booking (12–16 weeks), every pregnant woman should have a blood sample sent for determination of ABO and RhD group, and testing for red cell alloantibodies which may be directed against paternal blood group antigens

- Where a clinically significant antibody capable of causing HDN, particularly anti-D, anti-c or anti-K, is present in a maternal sample, determining the father's phenotype provides useful information to predict the likelihood of a fetus carrying the relevant red cell antigen. The complexities of paternal testing and the potential for misidentification of the father need to be acknowledged.

- Antenatal patients with anti D, anti c or anti K should have repeat testing regularly throughout the second trimester to monitor the antibody concentration

- All other patients should be retested at 28–30 weeks: prior to administration of RAADP (or up to 34 weeks for RhD positive patients with no antibodies) as later development of antibodies or increase in antibody concentration may occur

- If clinically significant antibodies are detected in pregnancy, specialist advice should be requested to ensure optimal timing of subsequent testing and intervention

Indications for anti-D immunoglobulin in a mother who is RhD negative

- Routine antenatal prophylaxis at 28 and 34 weeks (RAADP)
- **Delivery of RhD positive infant**
- Therapeutic termination of pregnancy:
  - all non-sensitised RhD negative women having medical or surgical therapeutic termination of pregnancy regardless of gestation
- Threatened abortion:
  - any after 12 weeks
  - prior to 12 weeks if bleeding is heavy or associated with abdominal pain particularly if approaching 12 weeks gestation
  - where bleeding continues intermittently after 12 weeks gestation anti D should be given at 6-weekly intervals
- Spontaneous abortion:
  - any occurring after 12 weeks gestation
  - any prior to 12 weeks requiring instrumentation (e.g. dilatation and curettage)

Other potentially sensitising events (PSEs)

- Invasive prenatal diagnosis (e.g. amniocentesis)
- Other intrauterine procedures
- Antepartum haemorrhage (APH)
- External cephalic version
- Closed abdominal injury/trauma
- Ectopic pregnancy
- Intrauterine death

Anti D should only be given to *non-sensitised* RhD negative pregnant women

Dose regime for anti-D (UK guidelines)

- **For RAADP**: 500 iμ at 28 and 34 weeks
- **Following delivery of an RhD positive baby**: 500 iμ as soon as possible and not later than 72 hours; check maternal sample for remaining fetal red cells (Kleihauer test or equivalent) and give extra anti-D if indicated
- **Other PSE**: anti-D should be given as soon as possible (within 72 hours) if the woman is RhD negative and has not already developed anti-D
- Prophylaxis is less effective if given later but may be of some value if given up to 10 days after the event
- **Dosage for PSE**
  - 250 iμ for events occurring before 20 weeks
  - 500 iμ after 20 weeks (this dose will clear up to 4 ml of fetal red cells from the maternal circulation)

Other countries employ alternative regimes using a dose unit of 1250 or 1500 iμ

For RAADP, regimes used are:

- single dose at 28 weeks
- at 28 and 34 weeks

The larger dose unit may also be used:

- at delivery
- for any potentially sensitising event (PSE)

Some hospitals in the UK use the single large-dose RAADP regime

Licensed anti-D products in 1250 or 1500 iμ dose units are available in the UK and should be used according to the manufacturer's instructions

www.rcog.org.uk   **www.nice.org.uk**

Management of HDN: refer early to a specialist unit

Patients with potentially severe HDN should be referred to a specialist unit for monitoring and management. The referral should be made before 20 weeks in those women who have had a previously affected baby. Affected neonates should be delivered in a centre which has access to specialist intensive therapy and experience in intrauterine and exchange transfusion. Delivery plans must also be communicated to the local haematologist and blood bank to allow them to provide appropriate support.

Transfusion of the newborn infant

Normal haematological values in infants (Table 20)

Normal blood volume at birth varies with gestational age and the timing of clamping of the cord. In term infants the average blood volume is 80 ml/kg (range 50–100 ml/kg) and in pre-term infants it is higher at 106 ml/kg (range of 85–143 ml/kg). Clotting times in neonates are prolonged compared to adult values, particularly in very low birth weight babies. At birth, activities of the vitamin K-dependent factors are 40–50% of those in normal adults depending on gestation; other factors, including fibrinogen, factor V, factor VIII and factor XIII, are in the normal range for adults.

Normal values for pre-term infants depend on gestational age. The normal values for Hb vary during infancy and childhood, with a nadir in Hb of 9 g/dl at two months of age increasing to 10–11 g/dl by six months of age. The levels of coagulation proteins gradually increase over the first few months so that coagulation screen results and coagulation factor levels reach adult values by 12 months of age. Results of coagulation assays are technique-dependent and therefore results should be related to the laboratory's own normal range.

Table 20 Normal haematological ranges for term and pre-term babies

	Term	Preterm	Adult
Haemoglobin g/l	140–240	140–240	115–180
Platelets × 10⁹/l	150–450	150–450	150–400
PT (sec)	10–16	11–22	11–14
APTT (sec)	31–55	28–101	27–40
TT (sec)	19–28	19–30	12–14
Fibrinogen g/l	1.7–4.0	1.5–3.7	1.5–4.0

Blood components for neonatal transfusion (Table 21)

A comprehensive guideline for neonatal and paediatric transfusion, together with a recent updating statement, is available at **www.bcshguidelines.com/**

Transfusion for neonates – principles (Table 22)

Minimise blood loss:

- Most red cell transfusions are given to replace blood drawn for monitoring: micro-techniques, non-invasive monitoring and avoidance of unnecessary testing should be used to reduce transfusion needs.

Minimise donor exposure:

- Neonates who may require several red cell transfusions within a few weeks should be allocated to a 'paedipak' system, where one donation is divided into four to eight small packs that can be used for sequential transfusions over the shelf life of the red cells (five weeks). By this means, the number of donors whose blood is transfused to the neonate is minimised.

- Close liaison between the neonatal intensive care unit and blood bank is essential to achieve optimal use of 'paedipaks' and ensure that all babies likely to receive more than one transfusion are identified.

Use a local transfusion protocol:

- Units with a written policy give fewer transfusions than those with no such policy. Recommendations for transfusion 'thresholds' are, at best, a consensus against which neonatal units can compare their local practice. Table 20a is given as a starting point for developing a local guideline.

Table 20a Indications for red cell transfusion in infants under four months of age

Clinical situation:	Transfuse at:
Neonate receiving mechanical ventilation	Hb < 120 g/l*
Acute blood loss	10% blood volume lost
Oxygen dependency (not ventilated)	Hb < 80–100 g/l*
Late anaemia, stable patient (off oxygen)	Hb < 70 g/l

* Some neonatologists use a Hb of < 110 g/l as a threshold for transfusing oxygen-dependent neonates, and since there is no good evidence to support a particular threshold value, each neonatal unit should produce a written policy of its own, based on the nature of the babies cared for by the unit.

Equipment for paediatric transfusion

As for adult transfusion, infusion devices must be tested and shown by the manufacturers to be suitable for the transfusion of blood components. Syringe drivers are suitable for neonatal transfusion. Whatever kind of system or giving set is used, it is important that a suitable filter (170–200 micron) is incorporated. This is preferably situated between the bag and the syringe during syringe filling. For small-volume transfusions, specific paediatric giving sets with small priming volumes are recommended. Blood components can be safely transfused through small-gauge peripheral cannulas (e.g. 19 G) or central lines, including umbilical catheters. Check your own unit's policy before using these catheters for the transfusion of blood components, as some neonatologists consider they may increase risk of necrotising enterocolitis.

Table 21 Blood components for neonatal transfusion
www.bcsh.guidelines.com

Component	Volume	Infusion rate
Red cell		
Exchange transfusion		
(Plasma-reduced whole blood in citrate phosphate dextrose, haematocrit 0.5–0.6, ≤ 5 days old, irradiated (page 56))	80–100 ml/kg (for anaemia) 160–200 ml/kg (for hyperbilirubinaemia)	Depends on stability of the baby – discuss with NICU consultant
Top-up transfusion		
(Red cells suspended in saline-adenine glucose-mannitol haematocrit 0.5–0.7, ≤ 35 days old, 'paedipak' if likely to need repeated small-volume transfusions, irradiated if neonate had intrauterine transfusion)	10–20 ml/kg	5 ml/kg/hr
Emergency large-volume transfusion		
(Plasma-reduced red cells have been advised: BCSH guideline now suggests that red cells in additive solution should be considered)	10–20 ml/kg	Rapid infusion only for resuscitation
Platelet concentrate (Adult apheresis packs split into 50–75 ml)	10–20 ml/kg	10–20 ml/kg/hr
FFP (Pathogen reduced*)	10–20 ml/kg	10–20 ml/kg/hr
Cryoprecipitate	5–10 ml/kg	10–20 ml/kg/hr

Notes:
Cellular components supplied for neonatal transfusion should be CMV negative.

* UK Departments of Health recommend that FFP given to neonates and children up to 16 years of age be obtained from an area free of BSE and subjected to pathogen-reduction procedures.

Table 22 Blood components volumes and rates of administration for infants and children

Component	Volume	Rate
Red cell concentrates	Vol (ml) = desired Hb rise (g/dl) × wt (kg) × 3	5 ml/kg/hr (usual max. rate 150 ml/hr)
Platelet concentrates	Children < 15 kg 10–20 ml/kg Children > 15 kg single apheresis or concentrate (approx. 300 ml; actual volume on pack label)	10–20 ml/kg/hr
FFP	10–20 ml/kg	10–20 ml/kg/hr
Cryo	5–10 ml/kg (usual max 10 units – approx 300 ml)	10–20 ml/kg/hr (i.e. over 30–60 mins)

Notes:

Transfusion rates are based on current practice, are only for guidance, and will depend on the exact volume given and clinical status of the patient. For neonates and children, it is important to prescribe the exact volume and the time over which the transfusion should be given.

Exchange transfusion

Exchange transfusion has a high incidence of adverse events. It should only be conducted under the supervision of experienced personnel.

- Exchange transfusion is generally performed for hyperbilirubinaemia and/or anaemia, usually due to haemolytic disease of the newborn (HDN) or to prematurity.
- For treating anaemia, a single volume (80–100 ml/kg) exchange is generally adequate.
- For management of hyperbilirubinaemia, a double volume exchange (160–200 ml/kg) is favoured.
- Plasma-reduced blood with a haematocrit (HCT) of 0.5–0.6 is recommended.

Blood for exchange transfusion should *always* be irradiated if the patient has already had intrauterine transfusion (IUT). Irradiated blood should also be used in other neonates unless delay in obtaining irradiated blood would cause clinically significant delay.

Epoetin in neonates

Meta-analysis of controlled clinical trials has shown that epoetin, when given with iron supplements, reduces red cell transfusion requirements in the anaemia of prematurity. Epoetin is licensed for this purpose. However, the effect is relatively modest, with no real benefit in the first two weeks of life when sick infants are undergoing frequent blood sampling and are therefore most likely to require transfusion.

Dose: A typical regime would be 300 mcg/kg three times per week for six weeks starting in the first week of life. Oral iron supplements (3–9 mg elemental iron/kg) should be used as soon as tolerated (see local neonatal formulary).

Thrombocytopenia and platelet transfusion (Table 23)

The risk of bleeding is increased in neonates with platelet counts < 50 × 10^9/l. However, safe threshold platelet counts in term and pre-term infants have not yet been identified. Table 16 shows suggested guidelines for platelet transfusion in the newborn. Babies with neonatal alloimmune thrombocytopenia (see below) may bleed at higher platelet counts as the bound antibody may interfere with platelet function. Monitor platelet count closely and consider transfusing with HPA-compatible platelets if platelet count is falling or in the case of a previous affected sibling with a history of intracranial haemorrhage. Some neonatalogists use a threshold for platelet transfusion of 20 × 10^9/l in well, stable term and pre-term neonates. At present there is no clinical trial evidence to support choosing a platelet count of 20 × 10^9/l vs 30 × 10^9/l. Neonatal units should produce their own written policy.

Table 23 Indications for platelet transfusion in term and pre-term neonates

Platelet count < 30 × 10⁹/l [1]
In otherwise well infants, including NAIT if no evidence of bleeding and no family history of ICH[2]

Platelet count < 50 × 10⁹/l
In infants with:

- clinical instability
- concurrent coagulopathy
- birth weight < 1000 g and age < 1 week
- previous major bleeding (e.g. GMH-IVH)[2]
- current minor bleeding (e.g. petechiae, venepuncture oozing)
- planned surgery or exchange transfusion
- platelet count falling and likely to fall below 30
- NAIT if previous affected sib with ICH

Platelet count < 100 × 10⁹/l
Consider platelet transfusion if there is major bleeding and platelet count is falling rapidly

Notes:

[1] Some neonatologists use a threshold for platelet transfusion of 20 × 10⁹/l in well, stable term and pre-term neonates (ref 6); at present there is no evidence to support choosing a platelet count of 20 × 10⁹/l over 30 × 10⁹/l and each neonatal unit should develop its own policy based on the nature of the babies that it cares for.

[2] GMH: Germinal matrix haemorrhage.
IVH: Intraventricular haemorrhage.
ICH: Intracranial haemorrhage.

Neonatal alloimmune thrombocytopenia

Neonatal alloimmune thrombocytopenia (NAIT) may be thought of as the platelet equivalent of haemolytic disease of the newborn. It affects about one in 1100 pregnancies. Maternal IgG alloantibodies are formed against a platelet-specific alloantigen on fetal platelets inherited from the father. The maternal antibodies cross the placenta and may destroy fetal platelets and cause bleeding. The commonest alloantibody causing NAIT is anti-HPA-1a (80% of cases). This occurs in a mother who is homozygous for the HPA-1b (2% of mothers are homozygous for HPA-1b but only around 10% make anti-HPA-1a). The second commonest antibody to cause NAIT is anti-HPA-5b (15% of cases), which in most cases causes only mild thrombocytopenia. Unlike haemolytic disease of the newborn, about 50% of cases occur in first pregnancies.

NAIT can cause life-threatening bleeding *in utero* or after birth. The most serious consequence is intracranial bleeding, which occurs in 10% of cases and may lead to death or long-term neurological deficits. The most common presentation of NAIT is unexplained severe thrombocytopenia in an otherwise well term baby or in a term baby with an intracranial haemorrhage. A useful practical point is that thrombocytopenia due to NAIT or secondary to pregnancy-related complications or infection resolves within weeks (sometimes up to eight weeks in NAIT), whereas thrombocytopenia secondary to bone marrow failure syndromes persists. Advice from a haematologist about the management of NAIT should be sought as soon as possible.

Treatment
The condition is self-limiting and usually resolves within two weeks. Occasionally thrombocytopenia persists for up to eight weeks. Several transfusions of compatible platelets may be needed. Rapid treatment is required if there is bleeding or a platelet count < 30 × 10⁹/l and treatment should not be delayed while waiting for a laboratory confirmation of the diagnosis. Give platelets lacking the specific HPA antigen. Blood centres should be able to supply platelets, which should be HPA-1a and 5b negative. If these are not available, BCSH guidelines now recommend using platelets that are not selected for HPA status. Administration of high-dose IVIgG is effective in about 75% of cases. IVIgG treatment can also reduce the period of dependence on compatible donor platelets. Additional doses of IVIgG may be needed two to four weeks after the initial response due to recurrence of thrombocytopenia.

Use of fresh frozen plasma in neonates

The only indications for FFP in neonates recommended in the recent BCSH guidelines and supported by evidence are: DIC, vitamin-K-dependent bleeding and inherited deficiencies of coagulation factors. The conventional dose of FFP is from 10 to 20 ml/kg.

FFP should never be used as simple volume replacement for polycythaemia. It is not effective in preventing intraventricular haemorrhage in pre-term babies without evidence of coagulopathy. The UK Department of Health now requires that children under 16 years of age requiring FFP should receive pathogen-reduced FFP of non-UK origin (see page 64).

Section 7
Adverse effects of transfusion

Reporting

Reports of serious adverse reactions or events should be made to the SABRE (serious adverse blood reactions and events) online system which can be accessed via **www.shot.org.uk/** See this site or **www.mhra.gov.uk** for guidance on reporting.

Acute life-threatening complications of transfusion

These are: acute haemolytic transfusion reaction; reaction to infusion of a bacterially contaminated unit; transfusion-related acute-lung injury (TRALI); acute fluid overload and severe allergic reaction or anaphylaxis. Serious or life-threatening acute reactions are rare but new symptoms or signs that appear while a patient is being transfused must be taken seriously as they may be the first warnings of a serious reaction. It can be difficult to determine the type of reaction in the early stages.

Recognition and management of acute transfusion reactions (Figure 10)

Acute haemolytic reaction

Incompatible transfused red cells react with the patient's own anti-A or anti-B antibodies and cause an acute severe clinical reaction (see page 16). Infusion of ABO-incompatible blood is most commonly due to errors in taking or labelling the sample, collecting the wrong blood from the fridge, or failure to carry out the required checks immediately before transfusion of the pack is started.

If red cells are mistakenly administered to the 'wrong' patient, the chance of ABO incompatibility is about one in three. The reaction is usually most severe if group A red cells are infused to a group O patient. Even a few millilitres of ABO incompatible blood may cause symptoms within a few minutes that will be noticed by a conscious patient (see page 61). However, if the patient is unconscious or cannot communicate, the first signs of the reaction may be bleeding, tachycardia, hypotension or hypertension. Acute haemolysis may also occur following infusion of plasma-rich components, usually platelets or FFP, containing high-titre anti-red- cell antibodies, usually anti A or B.

Management: Stop the transfusion. Maintain venous access. Resuscitate with crystalloid fluid. Consider inotrope support if hypotension is prolonged. Take blood cultures and samples for culture from component pack. Inform the blood bank. Seek urgent critical care and haematology advice. Admit to ICU if possible.

Infusion of a blood pack contaminated by bacteria

Likely to cause a very severe acute reaction with rapid onset of hyper- or hypotension, rigors and collapse. The signs and symptoms may be similar to acute haemolytic transfusion reactions or severe acute allergic reactions. Bacterial contamination of blood components is rare, but is more often reported with platelet concentrates (stored at 22°C) than with red cells (stored at 4–6°C). Examination of the pack (discoloration. smell and gram stain) may rapidly confirm the diagnosis. Organisms associated with contamination include *Staphylococcus epidermidis*, *Staphylococcus aureus*, *Bacillus cereus*, Group B streptococci, *E. coli*, *Pseudomonas* species and other gram-negative organisms.

Management: As for acute haemolytic reaction, and administer a combination of antibiotics that will be active against the range of bacteria that may be involved. In the absence of expert microbiology advice it would generally be appropriate to follow the local protocol for antibiotic management of sepsis in neutropenic patients. If this is not available, a combination of the following antibiotics may be considered to provide activity against gram-positive and gram-negative bacteria:

Gram-negative bacteria

Piperacillin/tazobactam (Tazocin) 4.5 g tds iv *or*

Ceftriaxone 1 g once daily iv (2 g if 'severe' infection) *or*

Meropenem 1 g tds iv

Gram-positive bacteria including most MRSA

Teicoplanin 400 mg bd iv × 2 doses then once daily (non-nephrotoxic)

Vancomycin – 1 g bd iv then adjusted according to levels – equally effective but potentially adds to any renal impairment

Ceftriaxone/teicoplanin has the advantages of once daily dosing, low renal toxicity

Transfusion-related acute-lung injury (TRALI)

Typically within six hours of a transfusion, the patient develops breathlessness and non-productive cough. The chest X-ray characteristically shows bilateral nodular infiltrates in a batwing pattern, typical of acute respiratory distress syndrome. Loss of circulating volume and hypotension are common. The patient may or may not have fever or chills. Monocytopenia or neutropenia may be seen.

Differential diagnosis: It may be very difficult to distinguish TRALI from other non cardiogenic pulmonary oedema or cardiac failure.

Management: Seek urgent critical care and haematology advice. Admit to ICU if possible. Treatment is that of adult respiratory distress syndrome from any cause. Diuretics should be avoided. Steroids are of uncertain benefit.

It is often found that plasma of one of the donors contains antibodies that react strongly with the patient's leucocytes. The implicated donors are almost always parous women. It is important to report any case of TRALI to the blood service so that an implicated donor can be contacted and, if appropriate, taken off the donor panel.

Fluid overload (transfusion-associated circulatory overload, TACO)

When too much fluid is transfused or the transfusion is too rapid, acute left ventricular failure (LVF) may occur with dyspnoea, tachypnoea, non-productive cough, raised JVP, basal lung crackles, frothy pink sputum, hypertension and tachycardia.

Management: The transfusion should be stopped and standard medical treatment, including diuretic and oxygen, given.

Note: Patients with chronic anaemia are usually normovolaemic or hypervolaemic, and may have signs of cardiac failure before any fluid is infused. If such a patient must be transfused, each unit should be given slowly with diuretic (e.g. frusemide 20–40 mg), and the patient closely observed. Restricting transfusion to one unit of RCC in each 12-hour period should reduce the risk of LVF. Volume overload is a special risk with 20% albumin solutions.

Allergic reactions

Anaphylaxis

A rare but life-threatening complication usually occurring in the early part of a transfusion. Rapid infusion of plasma is one cause. Signs consist of hypotension, bronchospasm, periorbital and laryngeal oedema, vomiting, erythema, urticaria and conjunctivitis. Symptoms include dyspnoea, chest pain, abdominal pain and nausea.

Anaphylaxis occurs when a patient who is pre-sensitised to an allergen producing IgE antibodies is re-exposed to the particular antigen.

IgG antibodies to infused allergens can also cause severe reactions.

A few patients with severe IgA deficiency develop antibodies to IgA and may have severe anaphylaxis if exposed to IgA by transfusion. If the patient who has had a reaction has to have further transfusion, it is essential to seek advice from the blood bank as there is a real risk of a repeat reaction unless blood components are specially selected.

Less severe allergic reactions

Urticaria and/or itching within minutes of starting a transfusion are quite common, particularly with components including large volumes of plasma, e.g. platelet concentrates and FFP. Symptoms usually subside if the transfusion is slowed and antihistamine is given (e.g. chlorpheniramine 10 mg, by slow intravenous injection or intramuscular injection in patients who are not thrombocytopenic).

Management: The transfusion may be continued if there is no progression of symptoms after 30 minutes. Chlorpheniramine should be given before transfusion if the patient has previously experienced repeated allergic reactions. If signs and symptoms fail to respond to this, seek advice from haematologist. Saline-washed blood components should be considered.

Febrile non-haemolytic transfusion reactions (FNHTR)

Fever or rigors during red cell or platelet transfusion affect 1–2% of recipients, mainly multi-transfused or previously pregnant patients. These reactions are probably less frequent with leucodepleted components. Features are fever (> 1.5°C above baseline), usually with shivering and general discomfort occurring towards the end of the transfusion or up to two hours after it has been completed.

Management: Most febrile reactions can be managed by slowing or stopping the transfusion and giving an antipyretic, e.g. paracetamol (not aspirin). These reactions are unpleasant but not life-threatening, but it is important to remember that the fever or rigors could be the first warning of a severe acute reaction.

Figure 10 Acute transfusion reactions

Symptoms/signs of acute transfusion reaction
Fever; chills; tachycardia; hyper- or hypotension; collapse; rigors; flushing; urticaria; bone, muscle, chest and/or abdominal pain; shortness of breath; nausea; generally feeling unwell; respiratory distress

↓

Stop the transfusion and call a doctor
- Measure temperature, pulse, blood pressure, respiratory rate, O_2 saturation
- Check the identity of the recipient with the details on the unit and compatibility label or tag

↓

Reaction involves mild fever or urticarial rash only

Mild fever →

Febrile non-haemolytic transfusion reaction
- If temperature rise less than 1.5°C, the observations are stable and the patient is otherwise well, give paracetamol
- Restart infusion at slower rate and observe more frequently

Urticaria →

Mild allergic reaction
- Give chlorphenamine 10 mg slowly iv and restart the transfusion at a slower rate and observe more frequently

↓ **No**

Suspected ABO incompatibility

Yes →

ABO incompatibility
- Stop transfusion
- Take down unit and giving set
- Return intact to blood bank
- Commence iv saline infusion
- Monitor urine output/catheterise
- Maintain urine output at > 100 ml/hr
- Give furosemide if urine output falls/absent
- Treat any DIC with appropriate blood components
- Inform hospital transfusion department immediately

↓ **No**

Severe allergic reaction

Yes →

Severe allergic reaction
Bronchospasm, angioedema, abdominal pain, hypotension
- Stop transfusion
- Take down unit and giving set
- Return intact to blood bank along with all other used/unused units
- Give chlopheniramine 10 mg slow iv
- Commence O_2
- Give salbutamol nebuliser
- If severe hypotension, give adrenaline (0.5 ml of 1 in 1000 intramuscular)*
- Clotted sample to transfusion laboratory
- Saline wash future components
(* equivalent to 0.5 mg im)

↓ **No**

Other haemaolytic reaction/bacterial contamination

Yes →

Haemolytic reaction/bacterial infection of unit
- Stop transfusion
- Take down unit and giving set
- Return intact to blood bank along with all other used/unused units
- Take blood cultures, repeat blood group/crossmatch/FBC, coagulation screen, biochemistry, urinalysis
- Monitor urine output
- Commence broad spectrum antibiotics if suspected bacterial infection
- Commence oxygen and fluid support
- Seek haematological and intensive care advice

↓ **No**

Acute dyspnoea/ hypotension
Monitor blood gases
Perform CXR
Measure CVP/ pulmonary capillary pressure

Normal CVP →

TRALI
- Clinical features of acute LVF with fever and chills
- Discontinue transfusion
- Give 100% oxygen
- Treat as ARDS – ventilate if hypoxia indicates

Raised CVP ←

Fluid overload
- Give oxygen and frusemide 40–80 mg iv

Delayed complications of transfusion

Delayed haemolytic transfusion reaction (DHTR)

DHTR is a haemolytic reaction occurring more than 24 hours after transfusion, in a patient who has been immunised to a red cell antigen by previous transfusion or pregnancy. The antibody may be undetectable by routine blood bank screening. However, red cell transfusion can cause a secondary immune response that boosts the antibody level. Antibodies of the Kidd (Jk) and Rh systems are the most frequent cause of such delayed haemolytic reactions. Features, occurring usually within 1–14 days of transfusion, may include falling haemoglobin concentration, unexpectedly small rise in Hb, jaundice, fever and rarely haemoglobinuria or renal failure.

Management: Investigations include haemoglobin level, blood film, LDH, direct antiglobulin test, renal profile, serum bilirubin, haptoglobin and urinalysis for haemoglobinuria. Renal function should be closely monitored. The group and antibody screen should be repeated and the units should be re-crossmatched using both pre- and post-transfusion samples. Specific treatment is rarely required, although further transfusion may be needed. The blood bank should be notified immediately and a report made to SABRE.

Transfusion associate graft-versus-host disease (TA-GvHD)

This is a rare but serious complication, due to the engraftment and proliferation of transfused donor lymphocytes. These damage recipient cells that carry HLA antigens. The skin, gut, liver, spleen and bone marrow are affected, usually one to two weeks following a transfusion, initially causing fever, skin rash, diarrhoea and hepatitis. The condition is usually fatal. Patients at risk are immunocompromised or those who receive transfusion from a first- or second-degree relative (due to the sharing of an HLA haplotype).

It is essential that all patients at risk of GvHD receive only blood components that have been irradiated to inactivate any donor lymphocytes.

Post-transfusion purpura (PTP)

This is a rare but potentially lethal complication of transfusion of red cells or platelets. It is more often seen in female patients. It is caused by platelet-specific alloantibodies. Typically five to nine days after transfusion, the patient develops an extremely low platelet count with bleeding.

Management: Seek specialist advice from haematologist. High-dose intravenous immunoglobulin (see page 44) is the current treatment of choice with responses in about 85% of cases; there is often a rapid and prompt increase in the platelet count. Steroids and plasma exchange were the preferred treatments before the availability of IVIgG, and plasma exchange in particular appeared to be effective in some but not all cases. Platelet transfusions are usually ineffective in raising the platelet count, but may have to be given in large doses in the attempt to control severe bleeding in the acute phase, particularly in patients who have recently undergone surgery, before there has been a response to high-dose IVIgG. There is no evidence that platelet concentrates from HPA 1a negative platelets are more effective than those from random donors in the acute thrombocytopenic phase, and the dose of platelets may be more important than the platelet type of the donor platelets. There is no evidence to suggest that further transfusions in the acute phase prolong the duration or severity of thrombocyopenia.

Iron overload

See page 37.

Infections transmissible by transfusion

Infection screening of donations

Donated blood units are tested for infective agents that are known to be transmitted by blood and to have the potential to cause significant disease, and for which there are practicable and effective tests. There are other blood-transmissible infective agents that are known to occur in the normal population, and therefore among blood donors, but which have not been associated with any illness, and further infections may emerge as transfusion risks. Every donation is tested for hepatitis B surface antigen, hepatitis C antibody and RNA, HIV antibody, HTLV antibody, and syphilis antibody. Tests for antibodies to malaria, T. cruzi and for West Nile virus RNA may be used when travel may have exposed a donor to risk of these infections. Some donations are tested for cytomegalovirus antibody to meet the needs of specific patient groups (see page 42). The epidemiology of infections in the population and among donors is monitored by the Health Protection Agency in order to inform future testing strategies for further risk reduction.

Frequency of transfusion transmitted infections in tested donations – estimated and observed (Tables 24 and 25)

On very rare occasions screening fails to detect the target infection in a donation. The risk of this can be estimated by calculation and also from the actual reported number of infections associated with transfusion. The estimated frequency of HBV, HCV and HIV infectious donations entering the UK blood supply in 2002–2003 is shown in Table 24. About three million blood component units are supplied (though all are not necessarily transfused) each year in the UK, so these estimates would predict that about one donation per two years could transmit HIV, seven donations per year could transmit hepatitis B, and one donation per seven years could transmit hepatitis C. The number of transfusion-transmitted infections reported to SHOT is shown in Table 25.

Hepatitis B

Hepatitis B can cause severe disease, and although most infected patients recover without serious complications, in some cases infection persists as a chronic carrier state. Patients who are immunosuppressed (e.g. those with leukaemia, cancer or transplant recipients) are more likely to go on to become carriers, often with high levels of infection. Tests for hepatitis B surface antigen (HBsAg) are extremely effective; there are very rare instances, however, in which HBsAg may be undetectable in a donor who is actually infectious. The role of tests for HBV DNA is still uncertain.

Hepatitis C

Although many people infected with hepatitis C are asymptomatic, some develop chronic liver disease and some will eventually progress to cirrhosis or hepatocellular carcinoma. Serological tests to detect hepatitis C virus infection were introduced in 1991. An additional test for hepatitis C RNA was introduced in 1999. It is estimated that the current risk of a blood unit infected with hepatitis C entering the UK blood supply is about 0.05 per million (or 1 in 22 million).

Human T-cell lymphotropic virus types I and II

HTLV infection is occasionally detected in blood donors in the UK; usually these are individuals from countries where the infection is endemic or the female sexual partners of men from these areas. Only a small proportion (less than 5%) of those infected become ill, but infection has been associated with a chronic neurological disorder (tropical spastic paraparesis) and a rare, aggressive malignancy adult T-cell leukaemia/lymphoma (ATLL). These conditions may develop many years after infection. All blood donations in the UK have been tested for antibody to HTLV I and II since 2002. Four HTLV-transmitted infections have been identified in the UK since 1991, all of which received transfusions prior to the introduction of leucodepletion of all components in 1999.

Cytomegalovirus (CMV)

See pages 41 and 42.

Hepatitis A

Hepatitis A is caused by a non-enveloped virus that is resistant to current methods of pathogen inactivation of blood components. Transfusion transmission of hepatitis A is extremely rare. In the UK, there have been four reports of transmission over the past 25 years.

Human parvovirus B19

Human parvovirus B19 is a prevalent, seasonal, non-enveloped virus that is quite resistant to current methods for pathogen inactivation of blood components. It can be transmitted via transfusion. Clinically, infection is generally asymptomatic or causes mild symptoms, but it can cause aplastic crisis in patients with sickle-cell disease, thalassaemia, chronic haemolytic anaemia or red cell membrane defects. Infection in the second trimester can lead to fetal anaemia, death or malformation.

West Nile virus

A mosquito-borne flavivirus infection causing encephalitis. Recent seasonal epidemics have occurred in North America. West Nile virus can be transmitted by blood donated during the viraemic phase. During the epidemic season, donors may not give blood in the UK for 28 days after returning from an affected area unless a test for viral RNA is negative. There have been no cases transmitted by transfusion in the UK and no infected donors have been detected to date.

Treponemal infections (syphilis)

There have been no reports of transfusion-transmitted syphilis in the UK in recent years. All donations are screened for serological evidence of *Treponema pallidum* infection.

Other bacterial infections

Despite all precautions, bacteria may occasionally enter a blood component pack, for example in skin fragments arising from the venepuncture. To reduce this risk, the first 20 ml of the donation is diverted from the collection pack and used for all the screening tests. Bacterial culture of platelet units is also being introduced, because a transfusion contaminated with bacteria can result in fatal transfusion reactions. Platelets are more likely to be associated with bacterial complications than red cells. Skin contaminants such as staphylococci may proliferate in platelet concentrates stored at 22°C. Bacteria identified in contaminated red cell transfusions are usually strains that can grow in red cells stored at 4°C. Examples are *Pseudomonas fluorescens*, an environmental contaminant, and *Yersinia enterocolitica*, which may contaminate a donation taken during an episode of asymptomatic bacteraemia.

Malaria

Only five cases of transfusion-transmitted malaria (all due to *Plasmodium falciparum*) have been reported in the UK in the past 25 years. In the US between 1993 and 1998, transfusion transmitted malaria (by several species of plasmodium) occurred with a frequency between zero and 0.18/million units collected. Blood donor selection procedures, and in some cases tests for malaria antibody, are used to identify and exclude individuals whose blood could transmit malaria.

Chagas' disease

This is a serious chronic multi-organ disease caused by *Trypanosoma cruzi*, and is transmissible by transfusion. In the UK no cases transmitted by transfusion have been reported; a small number of such cases have been reported in North America. It is an important problem in parts of South America where the infection is endemic. A negative test for antibody to *T. cruzi* allows the acceptance of donors at risk of infection.

Variant CJD

Clinical features and epidemiology
Variant CJD (vCJD) was identified in 1996. It is a transmissible spongiform encephalopathy (TSE) that is thought to be caused by the same agent as bovine spongifrom encephalopathy (BSE). This is an altered form of a normal protein called prion protein. During the period of the BSE epidemic, the UK population was exposed to the agent through consumption of beef. It is possible that there are healthy individuals who could be carriers of the agent. vCJD affects people younger (median age 29 years) than the long-recognised sporadic form of CJD. It also differs clinically, presenting with behaviour disorders, depression and anxiety, followed by sensory and coordination problems and progressive dementia. Survival from diagnosis is 6–24 months. To date about 160 definite and probable cases of vCJD have been reported in the UK, 14 in France, three in Ireland and single cases in a number of other countries. The eventual number of cases that can be expected in the UK is uncertain. Three possible transmissions of vCJD by blood transfusion have been reported. One of the patients died of unrelated causes.

vCJD precautionary measures taken by the UK blood and tissue services
Measures to minimise transmission by blood or tissues have been introduced as new information has become available. It can be expected that further precautions will be introduced. The measures summarised below have an important impact on both cost and availability of blood for transfusion.

- Withdrawal and recall of any blood components, plasma derivatives, cells or tissues obtained from any individual who later develops variant CJD (announced December 1997).

- Importation of plasma from countries other than the UK for fractionation to manufacture plasma derivatives (announced May 1998, fully implemented October 1999).

- Leucodepletion of all blood components (decision announced July 1998, fully implemented Autumn 1999).

- Importation of clinical FFP for patients born after January 1996, announced on 16 August 2003 and implemented by the end of June 2004, and extended to all patients under the age of 16 by July 2005.

- Exclusion of whole blood donors who state that they have received a blood component transfusion in the UK since 1 January 1980 (April 2004). Extended to whole blood and apheresis donors who may have received a blood component transfusion in the UK since 1 January 1980 (August 2004) and to any donors who have been treated with intravenous immunoglobulin prepared from UK plasma, or who have undergone plasma exchange procedures anywhere in the world.

- Exclusion of live bone donors who have been transfused since 1 January 1980 (July 2005).

- Exclusion of blood donors whose blood has been transfused to recipients who later developed vCJD, where blood transfusion cannot be excluded as a source of the vCJD infection and where no infected donor has been identified (July 2005).

- Further measures may include the use of processes intended to remove any infectivity that may be present in blood and the use of donor screening tests.

The single most effective way of protecting patients against both known and unrecognised blood-borne infections is to avoid the use of blood products or tissues unless there is a well-founded reason. This handbook and the associated website reflects the importance placed by the Chief Medical Officers of the UK on the appropriate use of blood and tissues.

Pathogen reduction and leucodepletion

The production of plasma derivatives includes physical, chemical and thermal processes to inactivate and remove pathogens. Chemical (e.g. solvent detergent) and thermal processes have reduced the risk of transmitting HIV, HTLV, hepatitis B or hepatitis C. Sterile filtration can eliminate bacteria and parasites. Cell-associated viruses such as CMV and HTLV do not pose a risk to plasma-derived products. Both plasma and cryoprecipitate may be subject to pathogen inactivation (page 10). Cellular blood components are not currently pathogen inactivated, but processes to inactivate microbial agents in platelet concentrates (using psoralen amotosalen-HCl combined with UVA light) have recently become available. These are not yet used in the UK. Leucodepletion reduces, but may not eliminate, the risk of transmission of pathogens that are carried by white cells.

Table 24 Estimate of the risk that a donation that is positive for HIV, hepatitis B or hepatitis C may enter the blood supply

Donations by	HIV	HCV	HBV
	Per million donations	Per million donations	Per million donations
All donors	0.22	0.05	2.20
New donors	0.50	0.19	6.7
Repeat donors	0.19	0.03	1.7

Rates of residual risk infection in UK blood donations 2002–3.
Calculated as described by Soldan K, Davison K and Dow B, *Euro. Surveill.* 2005 Feb 10(2):17–9.

Table 25 Frequency of reported serious hazards of blood transfusion in the UK

Event type	Events reported 1996–2004	Events reported per 100,000 components issued 1996–2004	Events reported 2003–2004	Events reported per 100,000 components issued 2003 and 2004
Incorrect blood component transfused (IBCT)	1832	7	787	12
ABO incompatible transfusions (all components – included in IBCT)	249	1	56	0.8
Death as a result of IBCT	20	0.07	3	0.04
Transfusion-related acute-lung injury (TRALI)	162	0.6	59	0.9
Fatal TRALI	36	0.1	9	0.1
Acute transfusion reaction (ATR)	267	1	73	1
Transfusion-transmitted infection (including bacterial)	49	0.2	6	0.1
Total adverse reactions/events	**2628**	**10**	**994**	**14**
Total transfusion-related deaths	**100**	**0.4**	**21**	**0.3**

Notes:

- Data reported to the UK Serious Hazards of Transfusion Scheme, 1996 to 2004.
- Data from unpublished UK studies indicate that individuals who receive a red cell transfusion in any year receive an average of four or five units. However, the distribution is skewed: most recipients receive two units, while a small minority receive much larger numbers.
- The risk of experiencing an adverse event is greater in recipients of greater numbers of transfusions, but is not a simple function of the number of units received.
- Over a period of eight years, 2628 events (not including 'near misses') have been reported to SHOT. During the same period, 27 million blood components were issued by the UK blood services. Using these figures, and the analysis of types of events undertaken annually by SHOT, the major risks of transfusion can be crudely calculated. Not all reported adverse reactions and events are included in the table.
- The total number of blood component units issued by the blood services to hospitals is used as the denominator.
- TRALI and severe allergic reactions (counted as ATRs) are some four to six times more likely to occur in relation to plasma and platelets than to red cells.
- The table does not reflect the number of patients transfused or the number of transfusion episodes.
- The causal relationship between the observed reaction and the transfusion is often not clear cut.

Appendix 1
Informing patients

Patient information leaflets are available from the UK blood services.

As with all treatments, a blood transfusion should only be prescribed when really necessary. The decision to give a blood transfusion to a patient should only be made after careful consideration. The risks of having a transfusion need to be balanced against the risks of not receiving one. Transfusion can save life and plays an essential part in the treatment of some conditions.

At present, there is no legal requirement in the UK to gain formal consent from the patient for the transfusion of blood products. It is, however, good clinical practice to discuss treatment options with the patient before reaching a decision to prescribe blood components. You should give the patient information on the benefits and risks of transfusion as well as any alternatives that may be available for that particular patient, such as oral iron therapy or autologous transfusion. It is essential that you provide this information in a timely manner that is understood by the patient, and that you ensure this information is understood.

A summary of some points that may concern patients is given below.

Why might a blood transfusion be needed?

Most people cope well with losing a moderate amount of blood (e.g. 2–3 pints from a total of 8–10 pints). This lost fluid can be replaced with a salt solution. Over the next few weeks your body will make new red cells to replace those lost. Medicines such as iron can also help compensate for blood loss. However, if larger amounts are lost, a blood transfusion is the best way of replacing the blood rapidly.

- Blood transfusions are given to replace blood lost during an operation or after an accident.
- Blood transfusions are used to treat anaemia (lack of red blood cells).
- Some medical treatments or operations cannot be safely carried out without using blood.

What can be done to reduce the need for blood?

- Eat a well-balanced diet in the weeks before your operation.
- Boost your iron levels – ask your GP or consultant for advice, especially if you know you have suffered from low iron in the past.
- If you are on warfarin or aspirin, stopping these drugs may reduce the amount of bleeding. Remember to check with your GP or consultant before your operation. (Please remember: for your own safety, only your doctor can make this decision.)

Are transfusions safe?

Almost always, yes. The main risk from receiving a transfusion is being given blood of the wrong blood group. A smaller risk is catching an infection. To ensure that you receive the right blood, the clinical staff make careful checks before taking a blood sample for cross matching and before administering a blood transfusion. They will ask you to state your full name and date of birth. They will then check the details on your identification wristband to ensure that you receive the right blood. They will regularly monitor you during your transfusion and ask you how you feel.

Appendix 2
'I want to donate blood for my own relative' (directed donation)

Information for clinical staff who may be called on to discuss this with patients and parents

The UK transfusion services generally discourage donation by parents, relatives or friends (so-called 'directed donation') for good medical and scientific reasons. Patients or parents may assume that there is a lower risk of disease transmission if the chosen person's blood is used rather than blood from the blood bank. However, published data show that blood from voluntary donors is in fact likely to be safer for the patient.

It is essential to discuss the following potential problems with the individuals concerned.

- The 'directed' donor may be inhibited from giving frank answers to questions about risk factors for infections. Studies show that directed donors do not have a lower risk of infectious disease transmission (based on positive tests for hepatitis or HIV). In fact, in some studies there has been a higher incidence of markers of infection in those who want to be directed donors than in the normal donor population. This is especially a concern when the directed donor is a first-time donor rather than a regular blood donor, as there is no history of previous testing.

- The donor may not have a blood group that is compatible with the patient's.

- Donors who are first- or second-degree relatives of the patient have a relatively high likelihood of having a similar tissue type – brothers and sisters have a 1 in 4 chance of being a 'complete match', parents and children of the patient will be at least 'haploidentical', i.e. matched for 50% of the tissue type. Thus there is a risk of the recipient developing graft-versus-host disease, which is a fatal condition (see page 62). For this reason all donations from related donors *must* be irradiated before transfusion to kill any remaining white cells.

- There are additional concerns when a mother wishes to donate for her child, in which case she should be aware that she may have antibodies to the baby's blood cells (red cells, white cells, platelets) and therefore that transfusion of her blood could cause the baby to suffer an acute or delayed transfusion reaction, respiratory problems, or a low platelet count.

- Transfusion of blood from a father to a young baby may also lead to a transfusion reaction, as the baby may have maternal antibodies.

- Older children may already have been sensitised against the mother's blood cells, as there is some passage of cells from the mother into the baby during pregnancy. This fact is less well known than the recognised risk of the baby's cells passing into the mother's bloodstream but also carries some potential risks. For example, if cells from the mother are transfused into an older child, there is a possibility that this will act as a 'booster' injection. The child may develop high levels of antibodies within a few days and break down the mother's transfused blood cells.

- Transfusion of a partner's blood to a patient who is or has been pregnant can cause acute reactions similar to those seen in the neonatal situation, as the woman may have developed potent antibodies to the partner's cells as a result of the pregnancy. In addition, the woman may develop antibodies after the transfusion, which may cause problems to the baby in future pregnancies.

- It is essential to make quite clear that if a directed donation is to be accepted, the donor *must* fulfil all of the criteria used to select normal volunteer donors, and that an individual who does not pass the normal donor screening processes will not be accepted as a directed donor.

Appendix 3
Patients who do not accept transfusions

Information for clinical staff

- Every patient has a right to be treated with respect, and staff must be sensitive to their individual needs, acknowledging their values, beliefs and cultural background.

- Clinical practitioners must be aware of Jehovah's Witness patients' beliefs in relation to receiving blood or blood products and of the non-blood, medical alternatives to transfusion that may be applicable.

- Jehovah's Witnesses are encouraged to carry a document at all times which details their wishes about medical care. Staff must take full note of this document. They must ensure also that the patient signs the appropriate form indicating his/her refusal to receive blood or blood components.

- Individual Jehovah's Witnesses may accept treatments such as dialysis, cardiopulmonary bypass, organ transplants or plasma derivatives.

- It is essential that each Jehovah's Witness patient who is competent is given the opportunity to discuss treatment options with a responsible doctor under a guarantee of strict clinical confidentiality.

- It is essential that any agreement to preserve total clinical confidentiality is strictly honoured.

Elective surgery

At time of referral (surgical out-patient department)

Check full blood count. Correct any haematinic deficiency (B12, folate, iron) and arrange further appropriate investigation.

If the procedure and the patient's condition are such that the clinician would normally request blood to be crossmatched, discuss with patient, parents or guardian which of the available and appropriate blood-sparing options or alternatives would be acceptable to them, e.g. cell salvage, acute normovolaemic haemodilution, erythropoeitin, fibrin sealant or albumin.

Six weeks preoperative:

Adults:	Oral iron
Children:	1–5 years: sodium feredate sugar-free 2.5 ml tid elixir 27.5 mg Fe/5 ml
	6–12 years: sodium feredate sugar-free 5 ml tid elixir 27.5 mg Fe/5 ml
10 days preoperative to 5 days post-operative:	Erythropoetin if the anticipated blood loss > 15–20% blood volume.
7 days preoperative:	Stop NSAID and aspirin.
3 days preoperative:	Stop warfarin where possible (see page 26).
At operation:	Use blood conservation approaches (see page 27), e.g. optimise anaesthetic technique – hypotension, hypothermia. Maximise haemostasis: surgical, antifibrinolytics, fibrin sealant. Conserve blood use: ANH, intraoperative, post-operative blood salvage.

Authors and reviewers

Section authors

J A J Barbara	National Blood Service	London
Vicki Clarke	The Royal Infirmary of Edinburgh	Edinburgh
Katy Davidson	National Blood Service	Watford
Moji Gesinde	National Blood Service	Leeds
Sandra Gray	Scottish National Blood Service	Edinburgh
Rachel Green		Glasgow
Lynne Manson	The Royal Infirmary of Edinburgh	Edinburgh
Helen New	St Mary's Hospital	London
Irene Roberts	Hammersmith Hospital	London
Clare Taylor	National Blood Service	London
Daffyd Thomas	Morriston Hospital	Swansea
J P Wallis	Department of Haematology, Freeman Hospital	Newcastle-upon-Tyne
Steven Yates	Musgrove Park Hospital	Somerset

Reviewers

Anne Benton	Morriston Hospital	Swansea
Susan Brunskill	National Blood Service	Oxford
Bruce Cuthbertson	Scottish National Blood Transfusion Service	Edinburgh
Marcela Contreras	National Blood Service	Colindale
Clive Dash	BIO Products Laboratory	Herefordshire
Brian Dow	West of Scotland BTS	Glasgow
Ian Franklin	Scottish National Blood Transfusion Service	Edinburgh
Paddy Gibson	The Royal Infirmary of Edinburgh	Edinburgh
Rick Heriot	The Western General Hospital	Edinburgh
Catherine Howell	National Blood Service	Oxford
Joan Jones	Welsh Blood Service	Pontyclun
Andrea Kelleher	Royal Brompton Hospital	Chelsea
Elizabeth Love	National Blood Service	Manchester
Sheila Maclennan	National Blood Service	Leeds
Lynne Manson	The Royal Infirmary of Edinburgh	Edinburgh
Elspeth Mackintosh	Scottish National Blood Transfusion Centre	Edinburgh
Alistair McGilchrist	The Royal Infirmary of Edinburgh	Edinburgh
Alastair Nimmo	The Royal Infirmary of Edinburgh	Edinburgh
Derek Norfolk	Leeds General Infirmary	Leeds
Jane Oldham	Western General Infirmary	Edinburgh

Denise O'Shaugnessy	Department of Health	London
Derwood Pamphilon	National Blood Service	Bristol
Elizabeth Pirie	Scottish National Blood Transfusion Service	Edinburgh
Jane Pelly	Scottish National Blood Transfusion Service	Edinburgh
Colin Robertson	The Royal Infirmary of Edinburgh	Edinburgh
Huw Roddie	Western General Hospital	Edinburgh
Anne Reid	Beatson Oncology Centre	Glasgow
Mary Rose	The Royal Hospital for Sick Children	Edinburgh
Colin Sinclair	The Royal Infirmary of Edinburgh	Edinburgh
Serge Six	National Blood Service	Bristol
Simon Stanworth	National Blood Service	Oxford
Dorothy Stainsby	National Blood Service	Newcastle-upon-Tyne
Audrey Todd	Royal Alexandria Hospital	Paisley
Marc Turner	Scottish National Blood Transfusion Service	Edinburgh
Jonathan Wallis	The Freeman Hospital	Newcastle-upon-Tyne
Tim Walsh	The Royal Infirmary of Edinburgh	Edinburgh
Douglas Watson	Scottish National Blood Transfusion Service	Edinburgh
Henry Watson	Aberdeen Royal Infirmary	Aberdeen

Glossary and abbreviations

Additive solution	Solution designed to maintain viability of cellular components during storage.
Allogeneic donation	Blood donated by another person.
Allogeneic blood products	Blood and blood components collected from an individual and intended for transfusion to another individual, for use in medical devices or as starting material or raw material for manufacturing into medicinal products.
Anti-D immunoglobulin	Human IgG preparation containing a high level of antibody to the RhD antigen.
Apheresis	A process in which whole blood is collected from a donor and separated into components. Some of these are retained and the remainder returned to the donor.
APTT	Activated partial thromboplastin time
Artificial colloid solutions	See 'Colloid solutions'.
ATD	Adult Therapeutic Dose. Usually used in reference to platelet transfusions. Refers to the amount usually transfused to an adult in a single dose.
Autologous blood transfusion	Transfusion to an individual of blood collected from him- or herself.
Blood component	A therapeutic constituent of human blood (red cells, white cells, platelets, plasma, cryoprecipitate).
Blood establishment	Organisation responsible for any aspect of the collection and testing of human blood or blood components, whatever their intended purpose, and for their processing, storage and distribution when intended for transfusion. Excludes hospital blood banks (EU Directive 2002/98/EC definition).
Blood products	Any therapeutic product derived from human whole blood or plasma donations.
BSE	Bovine spongiform encephalopathy. A neurological disease of cattle which is generally thought to have caused the incidence of vCJD in humans. See also 'TSE'.
Buffy coat	The granulocyte and platelet layer that forms between red cells and plasma when a pack of whole blood is centrifuged under suitable conditions.
CJD	Creutzfeldt–Jakob disease.
CMV	Cytomegalovirus. A type of herpes virus which is transmissible via transfusion and can cause infection in immunosuppressed patients.
Colloid solutions (artificial colloids)	Gelatin, Dextran, starch preparations.
CPDA	Citrate, phosphate, dextrose and adenine. An anticoagulant used for the storage of donated blood.
Cryoprecipitate	Precipitate produced after freezing and thawing fresh frozen plasma to precipitate high molecular weight proteins including factor VIII and fibrinogen.
Cryosupernatant plasma	Plasma from which the cryoprecipitate has been removed.
Crystalloid solutions	Saline, Ringer's lactate, etc.
DAGT	Direct antiglobulin test (Coombs' test). Sensitive method to detect red cell bound antibody.
DIC	Disseminated intravascular coagulation.

Erythropietin	A hormone produced by the kidney that stimulates red cell production by bone marrow.
EPO	Abbreviation for recombinant human erythropoietin.
Epoetin	Approved name for recombinant human erythropoietin.
FFP	Fresh frozen plasma. Plasma that is frozen within a specific time period after collection and stored in the frozen state until thawed for transfusion.
GvHD	Graft-versus-host disease. A serious condition in which allogeneic lymphocytes attack the tissues of the individual to whom they have been transplanted or transfused.
HAV	Hepatitis A virus.
HBsAg	Hepatitis B surface antigen. The presence or absence of this surface antigen is used to determine whether blood is infected with Hepatitis B virus.
HBV	Hepatitis B virus.
HCV	Hepatitis C virus.
HDN	Haemolytic disease of the newborn. A condition in which foetal red cells are destroyed by maternal antibody, usually anti D.
HIV	Human immunodeficiency virus.
HLA	Human leucocyte antigen.
Hospital blood bank	Any unit within a hospital which stores and distributes, and may perform compatibility tests on, blood and blood components exclusively for use within hospital facilities, including hospital-based transfusion activities.
HPA	Human platelet antigen.
HTC	Hospital transfusion committee.
HTLV I	Human T-cell leukaemia virus type I.
Human parvovirus B19	A non-enveloped virus transmissible by blood products and potentially pathogenic in some groups of patients.
Irradiated (blood component)	Cellular blood component treated with 25 gray (Gy) gamma irradiation to inactivate lymphocytes that could cause graft-versus-host disease in a recipient.
Kleihauer test	A method for counting fetal cells in maternal blood.
Leucodepleted (LD)	Blood component from which white cells have been removed by filtration or another method.
Massive transfusion	Variously defined as the replacement of one blood volume within 24 hours, or of 50% blood volume loss within three hours, or a rate of loss of 150 ml per minute in adults. In children it is usually defined as the loss of one blood volume within 24 hours, or 50% blood volume within three hours, or a rate of loss of 2–3 ml/kg per minute.
MSBOS/SBOS	Maximum Surgical Blood Order Schedule/Surgical Blood Order Schedule. Schedule of the normal quantities of blood ordered by type of surgical procedure, set at hospital level.
NAIT	Neonatal alloimmune thrombocytopenia.
NICE	National Institute for Health and Clinical Excellence (**www.nice.gov.uk**)
Pathogen reduction	Additional manufacturing step in making blood products, validated to remove or substantially reduce infectivity for infectious agents. Some viruses may not be reliably inactivated by current methods.

Plasma	The liquid portion of the blood in which the cells are suspended. Plasma may be separated from the cellular portion of a whole blood collection for therapeutic use as fresh frozen plasma or further processed to cryoprecipitate and cryoprecipitate-depleted plasma for transfusion. It may be used for the manufacture of medicinal products derived from human blood and human plasma, or used in the preparation of pooled platelets, or pooled leucocyte-depleted platelets. It may also be used for resuspension of red cell preparations for exchange transfusion or perinatal transfusion.
Plasma derivative	Licensed pharmaceutical product containing partially purified human plasma protein for therapeutic use. Prepared from pooled human plasma under pharmaceutical manufacturing conditions, e.g coagulation factors, immunoglobulins, albumin.
Plasma, cryoprecipitate-depleted	A plasma component prepared from a unit of plasma, fresh frozen. It comprises the residual portion after the cryoprecipitate has been removed.
Plasma, fresh frozen	The supernatant plasma separated from a whole blood donation or plasma collected by apheresis, frozen and stored.
Platelets, apheresis, leucocyte-depleted	A concentrated suspension of blood platelets, obtained by apheresis, from which leucocytes are removed.
Platelets, recovered, pooled, leucocyte-depleted	A concentrated suspension of blood platelets, obtained by the processing of whole blood units and pooling the platelets from the units during or after separation, and from which leucocytes are removed.
PTP	Post-transfusion purpura. Immunologically mediated thrombocytopenia following transfusion.
RAADP	Routine antenatal anti-D prophylaxis. A programme established to reduce the incidence of HDN.
Red cells	In this book the term is used for any red cell component unless otherwise stated.
Red cells in additive solution	The red cells from a single whole blood donation, with a large proportion of the plasma from the donation removed. A nutrient or preservative solution is added. The red cells from an apheresis red cell donation.
RhD	The RhD red cell antigen.
Saline	Sodium chloride intravenous infusion 0.9%.
Serious adverse event	Any untoward occurrence associated with the collection, testing, processing, storage and distribution of blood or blood components that might lead to death or life-threatening, disabling or incapacitating conditions for patients or which results in, or prolongs, hospitalisation or morbidity.
Serious adverse reaction	An unintended response in a donor or in a patient associated with the collection or transfusion of blood or blood components that is fatal, life-threatening, disabling, or which results in or prolongs hospitalisation or morbidity.
SHOT	Serious Hazards of Transfusion. UK-wide reporting system for adverse transfusion events and 'near misses'.
TA-GvHD	See 'GvHD' (Graft-versus-host disease).
Thrombocytopenia	An abnormally low platelet count which may indicate a bleeding risk.
TPH	Transplacental haemorrhage.
Traceability	The facility to trace each individual unit of blood or blood component derived thereof from the donor to its final destination, whether this is a recipient, a manufacturer of medicinal products or disposal, and vice versa (Commission Directives on haemovigilance/traceability).
Transfusion-associated graft-versus-host disease	See 'GvHD' (Graft-versus-host disease).

Transfusion-related acute lung injury (TRALI)	Acute lung injury following within hours of a transfusion.
TSE	Transmissible spongiform encephalopathy.
TTI	Transfusion transmitted infection.
TTP	Thrombotic thrombocytopenic purpura.
UKBTS	The United Kingdom Blood Transfusion Services, i.e. National Blood Service (NBS), Northern Ireland Blood Transfusion Service (NIBTS), Scottish National Blood Transfusion Service (SNBTS), Welsh Blood Service (WBS).
Variant Creutzfeldt–Jakob disease (vCJD)	A fatal disease which may be transmissible through prions transferred during transfusion of blood products from an infected donor. It is believed to be linked to BSE and affects much younger adults than CJD.
Viral inactivation	See 'Pathogen reduction'.
Whole blood	Blood collected from a donor before separation into red cells, platelets, and plasma.

Index

Page references in italic refer to information found in the Figures/Tables.
Page references with a 'g' suffix refer to definitions in the Glossary.

abnormal coagulation screen 24, *25*
   see also haemorrhage
ABO compatibility 16
abortion, threatened/spontaneous *53*
ACD (anaemia of chronic disease) 36
acidosis 28, *29*
additive solution 73g
   red cells in *75g*
administration errors 3
adrenaline *61*
Adsol 7
adult T-cell leukaemia/lymphoma (ATLL) 63
adult therapeutic dose (ATD) 73g
adverse reactions 59–66
   ABO incompatibility 59
   bacterial contamination 59
   febrile non haemolytic 60, 61
   fluid overload 60, 61
   graft-versus-host disease (GvHD) 62, 68
   high-dose IVIgG 43
   iron overload 37
   management 59–61
   monitoring the patient *22*
   parenteral iron 35
   records 18
   reporting 1, 59
   TACO 60
   TRALI 60
   see also infectious agents
albumin 2, *13–14*, 28
allergic reactions *see* adverse reactions
allogeneic blood products 73g
allogeneic donation 73g
allosensitisation 17, 38–9
Alteplase 31
anaemia
   cancer, patients with 36–7
   chronic disease, of 36
   chronic renal failure, in 38
   critical illness 32
   management 24, 35–6
   post-operative 27
   red cell transfusion 37
anaphylactoid reactions *see* adverse reactions
anti-D immunoglobulin 52, *53*, 73g
anti-fibrinolytic agents 15, 31
anti-inflammatory agents 25
antibiotics
   bacterially contaminated transfusion 59
antibodies 16–17
anticipated massive transfusion 30
anticoagulants 24, *25*
   see also coagulation factor concentrates;
      factors; haemophilia
antigens 16–17
antiplatelet agents 24, *25*
apheresis 73g
applied fibrin 15
aprotinin 15, 31
artificial colloids 73g

aspirin
   perioperative 25, 31, 67
ATD (adult therapeutic dose) 73g
ATR (acute transfusion reaction) 59–61, *66*
ATTL (adult T-cell leukaemia/lymphoma) 63
autologous blood transfusion 3, 26, 73g

ß-thalassaemia major 37–8
bacterial contamination 3, *61*, 63–4, *66*
   antibiotics in 59
blood
   administering 21
   administration errors 3, 59
   component 1, 5, 73g
      cytomegalovirus negative 2
      labelling 12
      leucocyte-depleted 2, 37
      mixing drugs with 22
      preparation 5–12
      therapy 5
   conservation approaches 24, 27, 28, 69
   donation 5
      allogeneic 73g
      autologous 3, 26
      directed 68
      unique number *11*
   establishment 73g
   expiry date *11*
   groups 5, *11*, 15
   labelling 5–6, *11*, 12, *21*
   management
      good 23, 24
      intra-operative 26–7
      post-operative 26–7
      preoperative 24–6
   ordering 17, *19*
   products 1, 5, 73g
      allogeneic 73g
   reducing the need for 67
   replacement of lost 67
   salvage 24, 27, 28, 69
   samples, taking *19*
   screening 62
   shortages 3
   tests 2, 5, 17
   variations in use 23–4
   warmers 21
Blood Safety and Quality Regulations 2005 1
bone marrow failure 39–42
BSE (bovine spongiform encephalopathy) 2,
   64, 73g
buffy coat 7, 73g

calcium-containing solutions
   dangers of mixing with blood components
      22
cancer
   adult T-cell leukaemia/lymphoma (ATLL) 63
   anaemia caused by 36
   hepatocellular carcinoma 63